Robotics in Skull-Base Surgery

Mohammed Maan Al-Salihi • Ali Ayyad
R. Shane Tubbs • Joachim Oertel
Editors

Robotics in Skull-Base Surgery

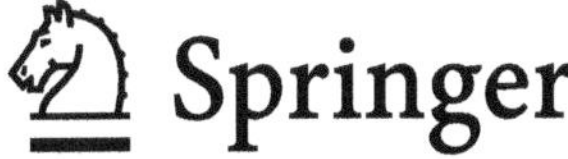

Editors
Mohammed Maan Al-Salihi
Department of Neurological Surgery
School of Medicine and Public Health
University of Wisconsin
Madison, WI, USA

R. Shane Tubbs
Department of Neurosurgery
Tulane University
New Orleans, LA, USA

Ali Ayyad
Department of Neurosurgery
Hamad General Hospital
Doha, Qatar

Joachim Oertel
Department of Neurosurgery
Saarland University Hospital
Homburg, Germany

ISBN 978-3-031-38378-6 ISBN 978-3-031-38376-2 (eBook)
https://doi.org/10.1007/978-3-031-38376-2

This Springer imprint is published by the registered company Springer Nature Switzerland AG
The registered company address is: Gewerbestrasse 11, 6330 Cham, Switzerland

Paper in this product is recyclable.

To my dearest mother, whose unwavering love and boundless support have been the guiding light in my journey. This book is a tribute to your strength and an eternal token of my gratitude.
Mohammed Maan Al-Salihi

To my mother, an epitome of love and wisdom, a rock of stability throughout my life, this book is dedicated to you.
To my wife and kids, who mean the world to me, inspiring me to be the best version of myself every day; this book is dedicated with all my love.
Lastly, to my teacher and mentor, Prof. Ibrahim Sbeih, whose guidance and support laid the strong foundation of my neurosurgical career; this book is dedicated in deep appreciation and gratitude.
Ali Ayyad

I would like to dedicate this book to my brother, Heath. Iron sharpens iron, and one man sharpens another.
R. Shane Tubbs

I wholeheartedly dedicate this book to my cherished family.
Joachim Oertel

Foreword

Mohammed Maan Al-Salihi and colleagues gave us a panoramic picture of neurosurgical robots in *Introduction to Robotics in Minimally Invasive Neurosurgery*. They surveyed the past, present, and future landscape from artificial intelligence (AI), Internet of Things (IoT), and virtual reality (VR) to "Nanorobots" and "Surgeon Supporting Robots." That compact overview allowed the interested practitioner—from medical student to physician (of all stripes) to senior neurosurgeon—to become "up-to-date" on neurosurgical robotics in a single sitting, if desired.

Less than 2 years later, Mohammed Maan Al-Salihi and colleagues serve us another intellectually stimulating view on neurosurgical robots in an anatomical subset of neurosurgical robots—skull base surgery. *Robotics in Skull Base Surgery* can also be read in a single sitting. However, this overview is composed of chapters that are more likely to appeal to practitioners of different stripes, for example, from transnasal approach of interest to the pituitary surgeon to cochlear implantation of interest to the otolaryngologist to radiosurgical robotics of interest to radiation physicists. Given the reader is more likely with this book to be more selective in chapters read than in the previous work, the repetition of basics and topics in some chapters is less likely to be noticed.

Skull base surgery "blossomed" several decades ago when the operating microscope and neuromonitoring allowed disorders (primarily tumors) to be approached. However, complications (e.g., lower cranial nerve impairments) despite the technological advances led to stereotactic radiosurgery as a viable alternative. Robotic techniques promise to make direct surgical interventions (as well as precision radiosurgical techniques) a viable treatment modality for skull base lesions.

Robotics in Skull Base Surgery covers the topic from history to present technology to speculation about future directions. The illustrations are numerous and informative, from line drawings to photographs of equipment and procedures.

In the final chapter "The Future of Robotics in Skull Base Surgery," the authors refer to Karel Čapek's 1920 play *Rossum's Universal Robots* (*RUR*). "Robot" in Czech can be translated as "slave" in English. In Čapek's scenario, humanity worldwide is undergoing a gradual decline—in both productivity and fertility—while the robots that (or who) the humans have created are evolving increasingly "human" attributes. The play ends with the humans being annihilated (their decline hastened by the revolt of the robots) and the robots becoming the latter-day "Adam and Eve" in a new global society.

Robotics in Skull Base Surgery describes ways in which robotics are transforming skull base surgery. Robots (AI, IoT, VR, and the increasingly sophisticated robotic instruments) in skull base surgery can be collaborators with neurosurgeons rather than the slaves of neurosurgeons. Unlike Čapek's *RUR*, all parties—the humans, the robots, and most importantly the patients—should benefit.

Nanotechnology and Smart Systems
NASA Ames Research Center
Moffett Field, CA, USA

Russell J. Andrews

Acknowledgment

I extend my heartfelt gratitude and special thanks to all the co-editors and contributors who have played a significant role in shaping this book. Your collective efforts and invaluable insights have made this project a success. Additionally, I would like to express my deep appreciation to Prof. Ayyad, whose steadfast support has been an essential part of my career, and to Prof. Tubbs for their invaluable contributions and unwavering encouragement throughout this endeavor. Your guidance and expertise have greatly enriched the content of this book.

Mohammed Maan Al-Salihi

This book is a testament to the immense dedication and perseverance invested in its creation. I extend my heartfelt gratitude to all who have contributed to the realization of this project, with a special acknowledgment to Dr. Al-Salihi for his invaluable role in its resounding success.

Ali Ayyad

I wish to thank my co-editors and especially, Dr. Mohammed Maan Al-Salihi who has spearheaded this publication.

R. Shane Tubbs

We gratefully acknowledge the expert support of our photographer Laura Gluecklich.

Joachim Oertel

Contents

Introduction to Robotics in Skull Base Surgery

1

Mohammed Maan Al-Salihi, Maryam Sabah Al-Jebur, Yazen Al-Salihi, Ram Saha, Md. Moshiur Rahman, and Sorayouth Chumnanvej

1.1 Introduction

The term "robot" was coined by Capek in 1920 to describe an automated machine used to replace human laborers [1]. Since then, there has been rapid progress in "robotics," where automated machines are designed to perform hundreds of functions in different fields, including medicine [2–4]. Present-day robots are designed to carry out not only simple tasks but also complex procedures requiring serial steps [2] via computer programming. These tasks can be automated, semi-automated, or passive, depending on the degree of human input during the robotic action [5–8]. In surgery, the use of robots has evolved dramatically from passive machines designed just to help surgeons perform certain steps more precisely, to advanced semi-automated robots requiring physician input only at certain points [9–11]. The

M. M. Al-Salihi
Department of Neurological Surgery, School of Medicine and Public Health, University of Wisconsin, Madison, WI, USA

M. S. Al-Jebur · Y. Al-Salihi
College of Medicine, University of Baghdad, Baghdad, Iraq

R. Saha
Virginia Commonwealth University, Richmond, VA, USA

M. M. Rahman
Department of Neurosurgery, Holy Family Red Crescent Medical College, Dhaka, Bangladesh

S. Chumnanvej (✉)
Neurosurgery Division, Surgery Department, Faculty of Medicine Ramathibodi Hospital, Mahidol University, Bangkok, Thailand
e-mail: sorayouth.chu@mahidol.edu

M. M. Al-Salihi et al. (eds.), *Robotics in Skull-Base Surgery*, https://doi.org/10.1007/978-3-031-38376-2_1

dramatic evolution of robotics in surgery has also enabled surgeons to perform not only local but also remote procedures via telerobotics [12–14].

The use of robotic surgery has increased dramatically during the past three decades [2]. A common surgical robot called the da Vinci surgical system (Intuitive Surgical, Sunnyvale, CA, USA) was designed to perform minimally invasive surgeries [15]. Since its Food and Drug Administration (FDA) approval in 2000, the da Vinci video endoscopic system has been increasingly adopted, especially in urology, gynecology, and otolaryngology [16–19]. This robotic surgical system has conferred several benefits: a wider range of motion within narrow corridors, motion scaling, 3D visualization of the surgical field, better comfort for the surgeons, and improved postoperative recovery [15, 20–23]. The da Vinci was the only commercially approved surgical system until 2020, when the FDA approved the Medrobotics Flex robotic system for use in different surgical fields, especially the head and neck [24].

Robotic surgery in neurosurgery dates back to stereotactic biopsy [25]. Thereafter, both automated and semi-automated robotic systems were developed and adopted for biopsy-taking from deep brain structures, deep electrode placement, placement of cochlear implants, and many other procedures requiring millimeter accuracy [26–28]. Four different categories of robots are used in neurosurgery: those designed for navigation and placement of depth electrodes, those designed for skull drilling, NeuroArm, and those (e.g., the da Vinci system) used to perform surgical procedures [25, 29, 30]. This chapter will focus on the last type, as used for skull base surgery.

1.2 Robotics in Skull Base Surgery

Although the rate of robotic surgery has increased dramatically in many surgical fields, as mentioned, progress in neurosurgery has been slower [31]. For example, there are relatively few data in the literature about the use of the da Vinci system in neurosurgery [31]. Notably, the da Vinci and the Medrobotics Flex robotic systems were not approved for skull base surgery [32]. This was because of their large size, long set-up time, and poor ergonomics, so it was not feasible to use them in the very tight corridors of the skull base [32]. Moreover, many studies evaluating skull base robotic surgeries were conducted on cadavers and/or animal models, and the results were discouraging [33].

Despite the slow growth of robotics in skull base surgery, neuroscientists are endeavoring to improve their development, enhance their adaptability, and make it possible to adopt them. Robotics fits the aim of this type of surgery perfectly, i.e., maximizing the exposure of a skull base lesion using the least amount of brain retraction [34]. This kind of surgery is challenging owing to the complex anatomy of skull base targets, their deep-seated location, and the proximity of critical structures. Robotics can provide more direct and less invasive access to the skull base than the conventional open surgical approach, avoid making cranial or facial incisions, and minimize brain retraction [32].

To date, the vast majority of skull base surgical procedures using robotics have been conducted to remove pituitary tumors [35–37]. Robotic-based surgery in such a procedure allows surgeons to remove the target tumors with extreme precision without injuring critical adjacent structures [38].

1.3 Robot Structure and Features

The only two FDA-approved and commercially available robotic systems for surgery are da Vinci and Flex [15, 24]. Neither was approved for skull base surgery; nevertheless, several studies have reported the successful use of the da Vinci machine in certain skull base surgeries [32, 33, 39–42]. To date, there have been no data about implementing the Medrobotics Flex robotic system in skull base surgery because it was only introduced into commercial use after its approval in 2020 [38].

The da Vinci surgical system comprises three components: a surgeon's console, a patient-side cart, and interactive arms [15]. The surgeon's console is typically in the patient's room, and the interactive arms are controlled from there [15, 20, 43]. The number of interactive arms varies according to the system model [15, 20]. They are used to grasp objects, dissect, cut into tissues, take sutures, apply clips, and perform different tasks with conventional surgical instruments, e.g., cautery. One arm controls a three-dimensional camera [15, 20].

The robots used for surgery (particularly endonasal endoscopic transsphenoidal surgery (EETS)) have different features, including their technique, interface, safety characteristics, tools for control, set-up time, and operative time [32]. The technique can be two- or four-handed depending on the size of the adenoma. The four-handed technique is preferred for large ademonas [38]. It entails meticulous collaboration between at least two surgeons [32]. One surgeon is responsible for holding the endoscope while the second performs the surgical dissections [32]. In long and complex procedures, this collaboration is usually challenging, particularly when rapid coordination is required to optimize the fixed visualization of the surgical field and the maneuverability of several surgical instruments in long narrow corridors [32]. Hybrid solutions have been provided to overcome this problem [44]. An endoscopic holder was developed, attached to the robotic system and controlled via a foot pedal. However, there are few data about their effectiveness because they have only been introduced recently [32].

The interface of the robot can be either cooperative or by telemanipulation [41, 45]. The collaborative approach requires the surgeon to hold and move the endoscope, as in conventional non-robotic surgery, but the robot maintains the position of the endoscope when the surgeon leaves it [45]. In the telemanipulation mode, the surgeon can control the endoscope's position via a joystick, foot pedal, voice, or head movement [41].

Many safety features have been incorporated into the robots to prevent accidental injury to vital neurovascular structures during procedures [32]. The most common of these features are an integrated 3D navigation system, loss of control mode, forced thresholds, vocal commands, and the ability to change the robot's orientation

[32]. The set-up and operative time also differ among robots, ranging from approximately 2 minutes to up to 30 minutes [45].

Robotics for skull base drilling have been described in the literature [25]. The most common are the computer-assisted design/computer-automated manufacturing (CAD/CAM) skull base drill [46], the replica study drill [47], and the drill described by Dillon et al. [48] These drills have given promising results, but none of them has been FDA approved to date [25].

1.4 Approaches to Robotic Skull Base Surgery

Skull base surgery is mainly carried out to excise neoplastic and non-neoplastic tumors or lesions originating at the anterior, middle, or posterior cranial fossae to minimize brain manipulation [49]. Each fossa requires specific surgical approaches for access, e.g., fronto-orbital and extended orbital approaches for anterior fossa lesions (e.g., congenital craniofacial malformations such as craniopharyngioma, meningioma, fibrous dysplasia, pituitary adenoma), and sellar, parasellar, petroclival, and lateral temporal approaches for middle and posterior cranial fossae lesions (such as meningioma and trigeminal ganglion schwannoma) [34].

Incorporating robotics into skull base surgery involves different approaches [42]. Not all the approaches used in conventional endoscopic skull base surgery, mentioned above, are used. Robotic surgery involves either single orifice approaches (transoral or endonasal) or multi-orifice approaches (combined transoral-transnasal, combined transantral-transnasal, or combined transcervical).

1.4.1 Endonasal Endoscopic Approach

The endonasal endoscopic approach (EEA) is the preferred choice in most skull base surgeries; endonasal endoscopic transsphenoidal surgery (EETS) has become the main technique for pituitary and sellar tumors because it is minimally invasive [38]. Less common EEAs include suprasellar, petroclival, and infratemporal approaches [50].

Several limitations have been reported in the use of robots in the EEA for skull base surgery. The commercially available endoscope provides 2D visualization of the surgical field; depth perception is critically important during surgery [50]. The ergonomics of robot use in the EEA are unfavorable because bimanual surgery requires the four-hand technique, the limitations of which have been described [31]. A third limitation is that the robots available commercially, e.g., the da Vinci system, were not designed to perform skull base operations. Their long and rigid structure precludes flexibility of motion and dissection into the tissues [51].

Successful experiments on 80 cadavers determined the characteristics of the EETS pathway and workspace for robotic design and development [52]. In addition, a navigator system with multi-information integrated tactics for surgery (MINITS) (Fig. 1.1), providing not only anatomical images but also the trajectories under a QR

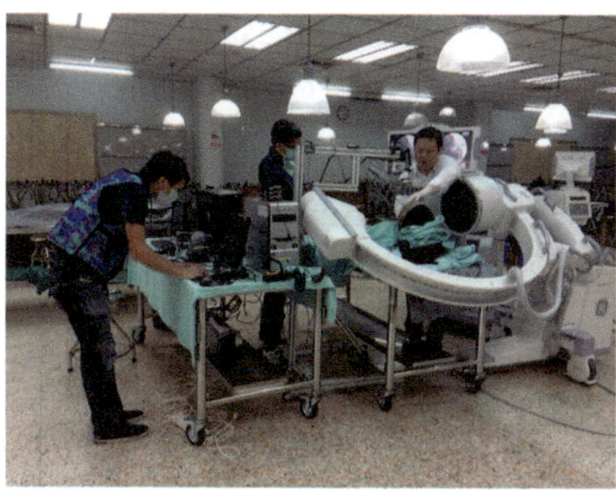
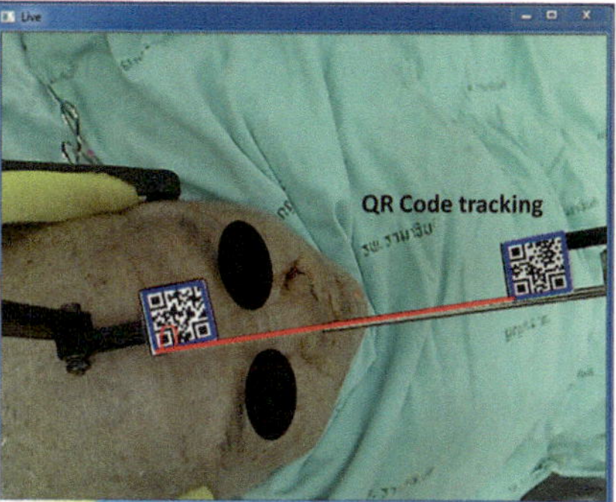

Fig. 1.1 The illustration shows the application of MINITS

code, is included for tracking the anticipated directions for neurosurgeons [53]. This is essential.

On the other hand, the robots allow 7 degrees of freedom and 90 degrees of articulation, which is not the case in endoscopic surgery, so the surgeon can reach narrow areas without tremor [54]. They are also superior to endoscopic surgeries in that they can suture the dura without the risk of cerebrospinal fluid leakage [50].

1.4.2 Transoral Surgery

Transoral surgery (TORS) is one of the most common approaches in robotic surgery, especially in the head and neck, to access the oropharynx, hypopharynx, and glottic region [55]. Since 1985 it has been proven capable of accessing structures from the fourth cervical vertebra to the sphenoid sinus caudally [56]. However, no attempts to use TORS in neurosurgery to reach the sella turcica were made prior to 2018, when Chauvet and Hans [31], in their three-stage study, used TORS on eight cadavers, computed tomography (CT) of 36 skulls, and 7 patients. They attempted to place the da Vinci machine behind the hard palate to face superiorly, unlike the conventional inferior-facing placement in head and neck surgeries [31]. Their findings showed that their innovative TORS held promise for reaching the sella region and pituitary tumors.

Not only was TORS successful in removing cystic pituitary tumors, but it was also shown by Malley et al. [40] to be capable of reaching the parapharyngeal space and infratemporal fossa and removing cystic neoplasms from those regions.

The TORS approach was reported to have several advantages over the widely adopted transsphenoidal approach. The side effects, especially rhinological, were minimal [31]. It allowed the surgical field to be visualized in 3D, not just 2D. The maneuverability of the surgical instruments was excellent, even in narrow spaces. There is growing evidence that TORS could be advantageous in handling pituitary tumors with large suprasellar extensions. However, the da Vinci system still has the disadvantage of being limited to cystic tumors [31]. Solid masses cannot be removed adequately even if they are well-visualized and reachable [31].

1.4.3 Transoral Robotic Surgery (TORS) Combined with Extended Endonasal Approach (EEA-TORS)

TORS combined with the Extended Endonasal Approach (EEA-TORS) was described by Carrau et al. [57] in 2013. They performed the technique initially on cadavers, then applied it to two patients, one with chondroma of the clivus extending to the second cervical vertebra, the other with a nasopharyngeal adenoid cystic fibroma extending to the infratemporal fossa and the hard palate [57]. The combined approach gave excellent results; successful total resection of both tumors with almost no complications and good postoperative recovery [57]. The advantage of the combined technique is improved visualization of the nasopharynx, infratemporal fossa, and the posterior skull below the eustachian tube level, which are not reachable by EETS. However, its success depends largely on the high level of experience of the surgeons performing the procedures, given the limitations of the robotics used.

1.4.4 Other Approaches

Other approaches for accessing the skull base via robots have been reported, such as the combined transantral-transnasal approach and combined transcervical approach, through which the authors successfully accessed the anterior fossa and sellar regions in several cadavers. However, this approach has not been attempted on patients to date [42].

1.5 Advantages

Compared to conventional endoscopic surgery, robotics has several advantages in skull base surgery [38]. It allows more detailed 3D visualization of the surgical field with a fixed view throughout the surgery, enhancing the accuracy of the procedure [58, 59]. Its considerable versatility enables the surgeon to perform tremor-free surgery, which is of the utmost necessity in narrow spaces with adjacent critical neural and vascular structures, as in skull base surgery [38]. Bimanual surgery is feasible using robots [58, 59]. Furthermore, the ergonomically designed surgeon's console allows the camera and all the instruments to be controlled fully [42].

Moreover, robot-assisted skull base surgery lowers operation times and therefore costs, especially for procedures requiring time-consuming drilling [25]. It reduces postsurgical discomfort and postoperative local complications (e.g., the nasal turbinate), shortens the hospital stay, and accelerates postoperative recovery [40, 60]. The da Vinci system also allows the dura to be sutured, which is not accessible with conventional endoscopic surgery, reducing the rate of infection and enhancing healing [25].

1.6 Limitations and Challenges

Despite the appealing advantages of robots in skull base surgery, several limitations retard their progress in this field. Along with their high cost, none of the commercially available surgical robots is designed to deal with the critical and delicate structures encountered in skull base surgery in such narrow surgical corridors [42]. The robots are large and rigid, making them challenging to handle through narrow spaces [38, 42]. The navigation systems are not fully developed, making tissue manipulation in the visualized surgical field suboptimal. Many other technical limitations still need to be overcome, such as the long set-up time for many machines and the lack of haptic feedback for surgeons. The robots lack the high-speed drills and suction devices crucial in surgical procedures in this region [58, 59]. The learning curve is also relatively slow, and the demands of collaboration in specific techniques (e.g., the four-handed technique) add to the challenge [32].

In addition, the literature provides few data about their efficacy and safety. Most studies have been performed on cadavers and a small number of patients with various conditions and in different centers with different levels of experience in neurosurgery [60]. Robots have proved effective only for cystic and soft pathologies; many skull base masses arise from rigid bony structures [25].

1.7 Conclusions

The use of robotics in skull base surgery is evolving, and robots have been reported to improve many of the limitations of conventional endoscopic surgery. Even though many advances are still required in software and structural development before robot use can be implemented in regular clinical practice, neurosurgeons should consider the advantages and disadvantages of robotic-assisted skull base surgery. Their decisions should be based on comparing the pros and cons of this technique to the conventional endoscopic approach in relation to each individual patient.

References

1. Nolte C, Ort T. Art and life in modernist Prague: Karel Čapek and his generation, 1911–1938. Am Hist Rev. 2016;121(2):667.2–668. https://doi.org/10.1093/ahr/121.2.667a.
2. Nguyen PT, Lorate Shiny M, Shankar K, Hashim W, Maseleno A. Robotic surgery. Int J Eng Adv Technol. 2019;8(6 Special Issue 2):995–8. https://doi.org/10.35940/ijeat.F1303.0886S219.
3. Makhataeva Z, Varol HA. Augmented reality for robotics: a review. Robotics. 2020;9(2) https://doi.org/10.3390/ROBOTICS9020021.
4. Vicentini F. Collaborative robotics: a survey. J Mech Des Trans ASME. 2021;143(4) https://doi.org/10.1115/1.4046238.

5. Low KH, Guo S, Deng X, et al. Special issue on focused areas and future trends of bio-inspired robots "analysis, control, and design for bio-inspired robotics". J Robot Mechatronics. 2012;24(4):559–60. https://doi.org/10.20965/jrm.2012.p0559.
6. Cobb J. Hands-on robotic unicompartmental knee replacement a prospective randomized controlled clinical investigation of the Acrobot® system. In: Navigation and MIS in orthopaedic surgery; 2007. p. 284–96. https://doi.org/10.1007/978-3-540-36691-1_37.
7. Fürtjes T, Korff A, Follmann A, Benzenberg J, Schmieder K, Radermacher K. Line of sight optimization for a semiautomatic hand-held tool for neurosurgery. Int J Comput Assist Radiol Surg. 2011;6:S290–2.
8. Zhang Y. A foundation for the design and analysis of robotic systems and behaviors. ProQuest Diss Theses. Published online 1994.
9. Stewart C, Fong Y. Robotic liver surgery—advantages and limitations. Eur Surg - Acta Chir Austriaca. 2021;53(4):149–57. https://doi.org/10.1007/s10353-020-00650-3.
10. Voutyrakou DA, Papanastasis A, Chatsikian M, Katrakazas P, Koutsouris D. Transoral robotic surgery advantages and disadvantages: a narrative review. J Eng. 2018;2018(5):284–95. https://doi.org/10.1049/joe.2017.0409.
11. Truong M, Kim JH, Scheib S, Patzkowsky K. Advantages of robotics in benign gynecologic surgery. Curr Opin Obstet Gynecol. 2016;28(4):304–10. https://doi.org/10.1097/GCO.0000000000000293.
12. Boabang F, Glitho R, Elbiaze H, Belqami F, Alfandi O. A Framework for Predicting Haptic Feedback in Needle Insertion in 5G Remote Robotic Surgery. In: 2020 *IEEE 17th Annual Consumer Communications and Networking Conference, CCNC 2020*; 2020. https://doi.org/10.1109/CCNC46108.2020.9045432.
13. Adler JR. Remote robotic spine surgery. Neurospine. 2020;17(1):121–2. https://doi.org/10.14245/ns.2040088.044.
14. Abbou CC, Hoznek A, Salomon L, et al. Laparoscopic radical prostatectomy with a remote controlled robot. J Urol. 2017;197(2):S210–2. https://doi.org/10.1016/j.juro.2016.10.107.
15. Watanabe G, Ishikawa N. da Vinci surgical system. Kyobu Geka. 2014;67(8):686–9. https://doi.org/10.1097/01.bmsas.0000415356.65864.d0.
16. Food and Drug Administration. FDA Approves New Robotic Surgery Device -- ScienceDaily. Published 2000. Accessed April 26, 2022. https://www.sciencedaily.com/releases/2000/07/000717072719.htm
17. Koukourikis P, Rha KH. Robotic surgical systems in urology: what is currently available? Investig Clin Urol. 2021;62(1):14–22. https://doi.org/10.4111/icu.20200387.
18. Kara M. Robotic surgery in gynecology practice: current approaches. Pakistan J Med Sci. 2012;28(1):238–41.
19. Nakayama M, Holsinger FC, Chevalier D, Orosco RK. The dawn of robotic surgery in otolaryngology head and neck surgery. Jpn J Clin Oncol. 2019;49(5):404–11. https://doi.org/10.1093/jjco/hyz020.
20. Kim DH, Kim H, Kwak S, et al. The settings, pros and cons of the new surgical robot da Vinci xi system for Transoral robotic Surgery (TORS): a comparison with the popular da Vinci Si system. Surg Laparosc Endosc Percutaneous Tech. 2016;26(5):391–6. https://doi.org/10.1097/SLE.0000000000000313.
21. Yu J, Wang Y, Li Y, Li X, Li C, Shen J. The safety and effectiveness of Da Vinci surgical system compared with open surgery and laparoscopic surgery: a rapid assessment. J Evid Based Med. 2014;7(2):121–34. https://doi.org/10.1111/jebm.12099.
22. Lee HH, Na JC, Yoon YE, Rha KH, Han WK. Robot-assisted laparoendoscopic single-site upper urinary tract surgery with da vinci xi surgical system: initial experience. Investig Clin Urol. 2020;61(3):323–9. https://doi.org/10.4111/icu.2020.61.3.323.
23. Bric JD, Lumbard DC, Frelich MJ, Gould JC. Current state of virtual reality simulation in robotic surgery training: a review. Surg Endosc. 2016;30(6):2169–78. https://doi.org/10.1007/s00464-015-4517-y.
24. Medrobotics. Medrobotics Receives FDA Clearance For Flexible Transabdominal, Transthoracic Robotic Scope - Medical Product Outsourcing. Accessed April 26,

2022. https://www.mpo-mag.com/contents/view_breaking-news/2018-02-12/medrobotics-receives-fda-clearance-for-flexible-transabdominal-transthoracic-robotic-scope/

25. Kundu B, Couldwell WT. Robotic automated skull-base drilling. Neuromethods. 2021;162:135–43. https://doi.org/10.1007/978-1-0716-0993-4_10.
26. Wagner CR, Phillips T, Roux S, Corrigan JP. Future directions in robotic neurosurgery. Oper Neurosurg. 2021;21:173. https://doi.org/10.1093/ons/opab135.
27. Ahmed SI, Javed G, Mubeen B, et al. Robotics in neurosurgery: a literature review. J Pak Med Assoc. 2018;68(2):258–63.
28. Bagga V, Bhattacharyya D. Robotics in neurosurgery. Ann R Coll Surg Engl. 2018;100:23–6. https://doi.org/10.1308/rcsann.supp1.19.
29. Adjepong D. The technological advancement for planning, navigation and robotic assistance for skull base surgery. Surg Curr Trends Innov. 2020;4(3):1–4. https://doi.org/10.24966/scti-7284/100042.
30. Maddahi Y, Zareinia K, Gan LS, Sutherland C, Lama S, Sutherland GR. Treatment of glioma using neuroArm surgical system. Biomed Res Int. 2016;2016:1. https://doi.org/10.1155/2016/9734512.
31. Chauvet D, Hans S. Transoral robotic Surgery applied to the Skull Base. Pituitary Diseases. 2019; https://doi.org/10.5772/intechopen.81048.
32. Madoglio A, Zappa F, Mattavelli D, et al. Robotics in endoscopic transnasal skull base surgery: literature review and personal experience. In: *Control systems design of bio-robotics and bio-mechatronics with advanced applications*; 2019. p. 221–44. https://doi.org/10.1016/B978-0-12-817463-0.00008-3.
33. O'Malley BW, Weinstein GS. Robotic anterior and midline Skull Base Surgery: preclinical investigations. Int J Radiat Oncol Biol Phys. 2007;69(2 SUPPL):S125. https://doi.org/10.1016/j.ijrobp.2007.06.028.
34. Kennedy JD, Haines SJ. Review of skull base surgery approaches: with special reference to pediatric patients. J Neuro-Oncol. 1994;20(3):291–312. https://doi.org/10.1007/BF01053045.
35. Soldozy S, Young S, Yağmurlu K, et al. Transsphenoidal surgery using robotics to approach the Sella turcica: integrative use of artificial intelligence, realistic motion tracking and telesurgery. Clin Neurol Neurosurg. 2020;197:197. https://doi.org/10.1016/j.clineuro.2020.106152.
36. Scraton RA, Liebelt B, Takashima M, Britz GW. Robotic exoscopic resection of pituitary tumors, vol. 79. J Neurol Surgery: Part B Skull Base; 2018. p. 79.
37. Obando M, Liem L, Madauss W, Morita M, Robinson B. Robotic surgery in pituitary tumors. Oper Tech Otolaryngol - Head Neck Surg. 2004;15(2):147–9. https://doi.org/10.1016/j.otot.2004.02.009.
38. Muñoz VF, Garcia-Morales I, Fraile-Marinero JC, et al. Collaborative robotic assistant platform for endonasal surgery: preliminary in-vitro trials. Sensors. 2021;21(7) https://doi.org/10.3390/s21072320.
39. Dallan I, Castelnuovo P, Seccia V, et al. Combined transnasal transcervical robotic dissection of posterior skull base: feasibility in a cadaveric model. Rhinology. 2012;50(2):165–70. https://doi.org/10.4193/rhin11.117.
40. O'Malley BW, Weinstein GS. Robotic skull base surgery: preclinical investigations to human clinical application. Arch Otolaryngol - Head Neck Surg. 2007;133(12):1215–9. https://doi.org/10.1001/archotol.133.12.1215.
41. Trévillot V, Sobral R, Dombre E, Poignet P, Herman B, Crampette L. Innovative endoscopic sino-nasal and anterior skull base robotics. Int J Comput Assist Radiol Surg. 2013;8(6):977–87. https://doi.org/10.1007/s11548-013-0839-1.
42. Heuermann M, Michael AP, Crosby DL. Robotic Skull Base Surgery. Otolaryngol Clin N Am. 2020;53(6):1077–89. https://doi.org/10.1016/j.otc.2020.07.015.
43. Fernandez-Nogueras Jimenez FJ, Segura Fernandez-Nogueras M, Jouma Katati M, Arraez Sanchez MÁ, Roda Murillo O, Sánchez MI. Applicability of the da Vinci robotic system in the skull base surgical approach. Preclinical investigation. Neurocirugia (Astur). 2015;26(5):217–23. https://doi.org/10.1016/J.NEUCIR.2014.12.002.

44. Zappa F, Mattavelli D, Madoglio A, et al. Hybrid robotics for endoscopic Skull Base Surgery: preclinical evaluation and surgeon first impression. World Neurosurg. 2020;134:e572–80. https://doi.org/10.1016/j.wneu.2019.10.142.
45. Bolzoni Villaret A, Doglietto F, Carobbio A, et al. Robotic Transnasal endoscopic Skull Base Surgery: systematic review of the literature and report of a novel prototype for a hybrid system (Brescia endoscope assistant robotic holder). World Neurosurg. 2017;105:875–83. https://doi.org/10.1016/j.wneu.2017.06.089.
46. Couldwell WT, MacDonald JD, Thomas CL, et al. Computer-aided design/computer-aided manufacturing skull base drill. Neurosurg Focus. 2017;42(5):E6. https://doi.org/10.3171/2017.2.FOCUS16561.
47. Lim H, Matsumoto N, Cho B, et al. Semi-manual mastoidectomy assisted by human-robot collaborative control - a temporal bone replica study. Auris Nasus Larynx. 2016;43(2):161–5. https://doi.org/10.1016/j.anl.2015.08.008.
48. Dillon NP, Balachandran R, Siebold MA, Webster RJ, Wanna GB, Labadie RF. Cadaveric testing of robot-assisted access to the internal Auditory Canal for vestibular schwannoma removal. Otol Neurotol. 2017;38(3):441–7. https://doi.org/10.1097/MAO.0000000000001324.
49. Sekhar LN, Juric-Sekhar G, Qazi Z, et al. The future of Skull Base Surgery: a view through tinted glasses. World Neurosurg. 2020;142:29–42. https://doi.org/10.1016/j.wneu.2020.06.172.
50. Kupferman ME, Hanna E. Robotic Surgery of the Skull Base. Otolaryngol Clin N Am. 2014;47(3):415–23. https://doi.org/10.1016/j.otc.2014.02.004.
51. Campbell RG. Robotic surgery of the anterior skull base. Int Forum Allergy Rhinol. 2019;9(12):1508–14. https://doi.org/10.1002/alr.22435.
52. Chumnanvej S, Chalongwongse S, Pillai BM, Suthakorn J. Pathway and workspace study of Endonasal Endoscopic Transsphenoidal (EET) approach in cadavers. Int J Surg Open. 2019;16:22–8.
53. Chumnanvej S, Pillai BM, Chalongwongse S, Suthakorn J. Endonasal endoscopic transsphenoidal approach robot prototype: A cadaveric trial. Asian J Surg. 2021;44(1):345–51. https://doi.org/10.1016/j.asjsur.2020.08.011. Epub 2020 Sep 18
54. Burgner J, Swaney PJ, Rucker DC, et al. A bimanual teleoperated system for endonasal skull base surgery. In: *IEEE International Conference on Intelligent Robots and Systems*; 2011. p. 2517–23. https://doi.org/10.1109/IROS.2011.6048276.
55. Rao KN, Gangiti KK. Transoral robotic Surgery. Indian J Surg Oncol. 2021;12(4):847–53. https://doi.org/10.1007/s13193-021-01443-0.
56. Crockard HA. The transoral approach to the base of the brain and upper cervical cord. Ann R Coll Surg Engl. 1985;67(5):321–5.
57. Carrau RL, Prevedello DM, De Lara D, Durmus K, Ozer E. Combined transoral robotic surgery and endoscopic endonasal approach for the resection of extensive malignancies of the skull base. Head Neck. 2013;35(11):E351. https://doi.org/10.1002/hed.23238.
58. Hachem RA, Rangarajan S, Beer-Furlan A, Prevedello D, Ozer E, Carrau RL. The role of robotic Surgery in Sinonasal and ventral Skull Base malignancy. Otolaryngol Clin N Am. 2017;50(2):385–95. https://doi.org/10.1016/j.otc.2016.12.012.
59. Castelnuovo P, Dallan I, Battaglia P, Bignami M. Endoscopic endonasal skull base surgery: past, present and future. Eur Arch Oto-Rhino-Laryngol. 2010;267(5):649–63. https://doi.org/10.1007/s00405-009-1196-0.
60. Emerging Role of Robotics in Skull Base Surgery. Accessed April 25, 2022. https://www.pulsus.com/scholarly-articles/emerging-role-of-robotics-in-skull-base-surgery-8738.html

Robotics in Transoral Approaches of the Skull Base

2

Joachim Oertel and Jason Degiannis

2.1 Introduction

Over the last few decades, the use of minimally invasive surgical procedures has expanded. These include endoscopic or laparoscopic surgery, which was initially applied to the abdominal and pelvic cavities and later to other anatomical areas. Its popularity grew because it used a limited number of small entry points. Coupled with the shorter in-hospital stay and faster recovery, this made it a more popular choice than open surgery for many indications.

Minimally invasive surgery was further advanced by the inclusion of robotic technology. The primary advantage of robotic surgery over classical endoscopic-navigated approaches is the detailed visualization of the operative field provided by three-dimensional (3D) technology; 3D imaging is not yet widely used in endoscopic surgery. Additionally, motion scaling and tremor filtration software enables the surgeon to maintain precision while performing operations that require maximum dexterity. Furthermore, better lighting provided by a dual source, together with automatic maintenance of instrumental positioning and position memory for instrument changes, is greatly advantageous for the surgeon in a robotic procedure.

2.1.1 Evolution of Robotic Surgery

To date, robotic technology has mainly been applied to the lungs, the heart, and the urological, gynecological and digestive systems. Specifically, regarding neurosurgical operative procedures, minimally invasive surgery has long been applied to the

J. Oertel (✉) · J. Degiannis
Klinik für Neurochirurgie, Universitätsklinikum des Saarlandes, Medizinische Fakultät, Universität des Saarlandes, Homburg, Germany
e-mail: Joachim.Oertel@uks.eu; Jason.Degiannis@uks.eu

M. M. Al-Salihi et al. (eds.), *Robotics in Skull-Base Surgery*,
https://doi.org/10.1007/978-3-031-38376-2_2

treatment of various pathologies including vascular malformations, a wide range of brain tumors, aneurysms, strokes, epilepsy, and Parkinson's disease as well as spinal pathologies. Many of these are frame-based or frameless stereotactic-navigated in application.

Endoscopic endonasal approaches (EEA) have become the "gold standard" for trans-sphenoidal, trans-ethmoidal, and trans-clival access to the base of the skull. Although these techniques have the standard advantages of endoscopic surgery, 3D imaging is still being evaluated rather than established. The trend is more toward the introduction of 4 K imaging than 3D. Thus, the technical drawbacks related to 2D vision persist. Also, the difficulty of spatial movement when both hands are used in fine dissections—for example, for dural fistula closure—within the narrow operative corridor remains a disadvantage compared to the more invasive classical open surgical dissection.

Considering the shortcomings of endonasal endoscopic techniques in accessing the base of the skull, a logical step was to use robotic surgery in an attempt to achieve more comfortable surgical manipulation while simultaneously using an alternative route of access to the sphenoid bone, avoiding potential rhinological complications.

A transoral approach to the base of the skull—more or less reserved in earlier neurosurgery for the rare indication of odontoid bone resection—was considered; there was already significant reported experience of robotic surgery on the base of the skull in conjunction with the treatment of otolaryngological pathologies. Over the last decade, a few pioneering publications described successful access to the base of the skull via robotic transoral surgery (TORS), aimed at training toward the treatment of clival and sellar pathologies. The current literature remains sparse but allows us to envision a potentially promising possibility for treating neurosurgical pathologies of the skull base.

2.2 Key Publications about TORS

In 2022, Pangal et al. published a systemic literature review spanning from January 1, 1990, to August 2, 2021, and identified all robotic systems used in neurosurgical procedures on the skull base. Cadaveric and human clinical studies were included. Only four studies were identified as relating to a robotic transoral approach (TORS) to the sella turcica [1].

In two of these studies, robotics was used by the surgeons on cadavers to assess the feasibility of transoral access to the base of the skull prior to operating on patients. At this point, it is worth mentioning that working on cadavers is more beneficial than virtual reality training, as it includes stereotactic elements that allow the surgeons to experience the pseudo–3D environment of robotic systems, thus allowing extended proprioceptive feedback of the tools to be obtained [2].

In view of the novelty of the transoral approach, it is useful to approach each of the four publications individually. It is worth mentioning that the da Vinci robotic system was used in all four.

The first published paper came from the Carrau et al. skull base group and was published in the journal Head and Neck in 2013 [3]. The authors reported two procedures carried out on two fresh cadaveric specimens and subsequently surgery on two cases. In the cadavers, the feasibility of combining transoral robotic surgery (TORS) with an endoscopic endonasal approach (EEA) was demonstrated by completing an oncological nasopharyngectomy with inferior and lateral extensions to the area of the cranio-cervical junction and to the infratemporal middle cranial fossa.

The combined TORS and EEA surgery was then used on two patients to treat tumors that extended past the cranio-cervical junction. One patient had an adenoid cystic carcinoma extending into the sphenoid sinus and clivus; the other had a chordoma extending from the posterior middle skull base to the C2 level. In the authors' technique, the EEA was used to access the tumor at the C1 level, and thereafter the TORS approach was used to complete the resection at the C2 level. The operations were performed by cooperation between ENT (Ear-Nose-Throat) and neurosurgeons, and the outcomes were satisfactory.

In 2014, Fernandes-Nogueras et al. published their experience of an entirely transoral approach to the central skull base through the nasopharynx on two cadavers [4]. To allow extensive opening of the mouth, they used two large self-retraining retractors, one separating the maxilla and the mandible and the other the two cheeks. This was preferred to mouth gags as it provided better access to the oral cavity. The robotic system was placed cranially with the skull facing the patient-side cart, resulting in more maneuverability of the robotic arms. A 30° endoscope was inserted through, facing toward the soft palate, which was separated from the hard palate by sharp dissection. The endoscope was then inserted via the newly formed opening into the nasopharynx until the upper part of the choana and the posterior edge of the vomer could be visualized.

The mucosa of the posterior wall of the nasopharynx was then dissected with scissors, starting the incision at the upper left margin of the choanae, continuing to the upper right parts of both choanae along the posterolateral portion of nasopharynx, behind the posterior limit of the Eustachian tube, up to the boundary between the oro- and nasopharynx. The left posterolateral region was dissected similarly. Following this, the mucous membrane of the posterior wall was pulled down, together with the soft tissues, through blunt and sharp dissection. This enabled the vomer to be visualized on the floor of the sphenoid sinus.

Thereafter, the authors removed the robotic arm leaving the 30° endoscope inside to provide a clear view on a 2D monitor. This was because the bony parts had to be perforated, and the armamentarium of the da Vinci robotic system lacks a drill. A drill was inserted through the mouth and the outer wall of the floor of the sphenoid bone just behind the insertion of the vomer. The floor of the sellae, the bony covering of the internal carotid arteries, the bony coverings of the optic nerves, the optic chiasm, the planum sphenoidale and the upper clivus were drilled.

The drill was then removed and the robotic arms were reinserted allowing the viscera to be dissected at this level, i.e., the internal carotids, the ophthalmic arteries, the optic chiasm and the optic nerve, and tracts. The authors reported their experience with this entirely transoral procedure as most satisfactory. By "deroofing" the base of the skull to a considerable extent, they succeeded in obtaining an excellent view of the relevant structures thanks to the advantages offered by robotic surgery, as well as easily dissecting relevant anatomical structures at the base of the skull.

The third and fourth publications were by Chauvet et al. in 2014 and 2017. The earlier of them was a cadaveric study concerning transoral robotic-assisted skull base surgery in approaching the sellae turcica [5]. The latter was the first and only clinical study of transoral robotic surgical removal of sellae tumors ever reported [6]. A book chapter based on the experience of these two publications was published by Chauvet et al. in 2019 [7].

In total, Chauvet et al. performed 11 cadaveric dissections [4]. Two surgeons were involved in each dissection, a head and neck surgeon (Chauvet) at the console and a neurosurgeon at the side of the bed (Fig. 2.1). The head and neck surgeon performed the mucosal part of the operation, creating the flap of the posterior cavum mucosa, which corresponded to the mucosa covering the sphenoidal rostrum anteriorly and inferiorly up to the opening of the sphenoid sinus. The sphenoid sinus was then drilled by the neurosurgeon, who controlled the progress of his procedure by watching on his 2D flat panel screen. Assistance for this was also offered by the head and neck surgeon sitting at the console and carrying out intraoperative control with the 3D view provided by the robot. An extensive view of the sellae turcica was provided by enlarging the sphenoid sinus with a Kerrison punch [7].

The group also performed an anatomical study to establish how much opening of the mouth is sufficient for a TORS to be performed without particular difficulty in positioning the equipment needed to approach the sella turcica. Patients with mouth

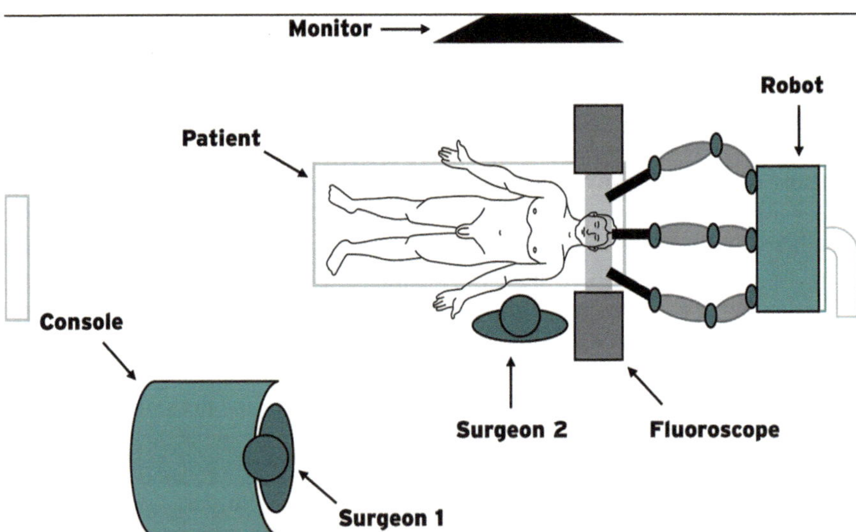

Fig. 2.1 Schematic drawing of the operating room set-up. Surgeon 1 is the head and neck surgeon working at the console and surgeon 2 is the neurosurgeon working at the bedside. Schematic drawing after the figure from Chauvet and Hans [7]

openings of less than 3 cm were excluded from the study. The authors studied anatomical criteria using radiological data from patients requiring a cerebral CT scan for neurological issues. The patients were asked to open their mouths as widely as they could during the CT scan, with no retractor. In summary, the authors defined, on a sagittal midline CT view, five points for each patient corresponding to strategic landmarks: the lowest point of the sella turcica, the most anterior and the most posterior palatine bone points, and the tips of the superior and inferior incisors. They also took CT measurements of four other distances between the previous points—mouth opening, length of palate, distance between the posterior edge of the palate and the sella and distance between the inferior incisors and the posterior end of the palate. The data confirmed that the physiological maximum mouth opening corresponds to an excellent predictive value for the feasibility of TORS [7].

Following these two studies, the authors proceeded with the only reported clinical study exclusively using TORS to access the base of the skull in four patients with cystic sella masses. As with the cadavers, the sphenoid sinus was drilled using a traditional endoscopic (non-robotic) drill, following which the operation was again carried out by the robot. Before the sphenoid was drilled, the angle of attack of the drill was also verified using lateral fluoroscopy, which had not happened with the cadavers (Fig. 2.2). The dura was then coagulated with robotic instruments and was opened using a CO_2 laser provided by the robot. All tumors were cystic and burst when the dura was opened. The sella turcica was curettage (Fig. 2.3). There were complications in two patients; one developed a CSF leak and the other had diabetes insipidus. The visual symptoms improved, and there were no symptoms directly related to TORS. The authors stated that the picture provided through TORS was more stable than that in EEA. They also stated that the TORS approach to the sella turcica could well facilitate resection of tumors even with significant suprasellar extension. Finally, they suggested that further studies should be conducted to compare TORS with EEA. Technological developments will further facilitate the application of TORS to the resectioning of sellar tumors [7].

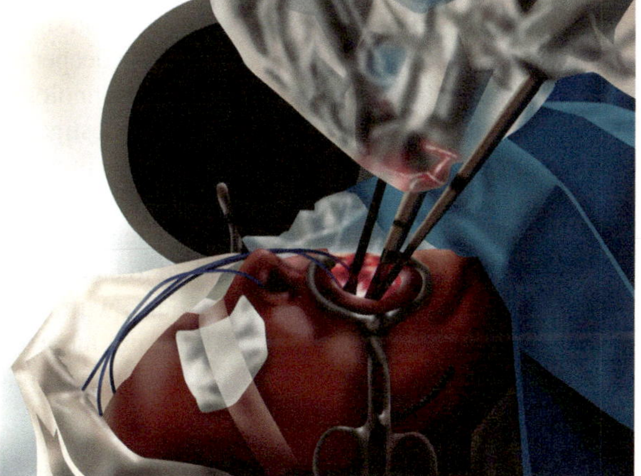

Fig. 2.2 Lateral intraoperative view. The three robotic arms stand in the oral cavity, which is opened with a mouth retractor. The soft palate is retracted using two rubber catheters introduced via the nose and pulled out via the mouth. In the background, the C-arm fluoroscope for intraoperative 2D lateral control. Schematic drawing after the figure from Chauvet and Hans [7]

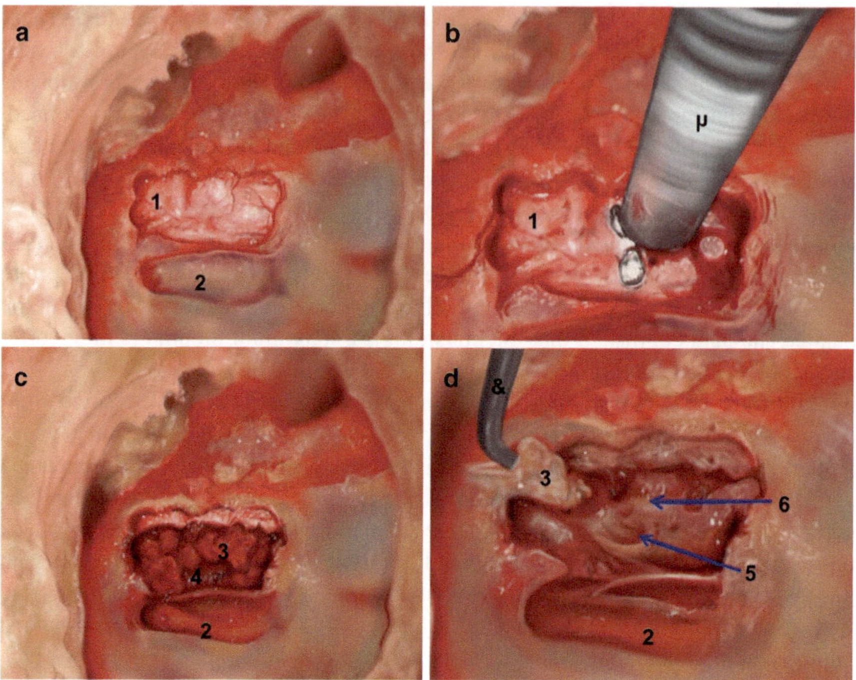

Fig. 2.3 Schematic drawing of the intraoperative view of a pituitary fossa dissection. (**a**) View after sellar floor removal. (**b**) Cauterization of the sellar dura with monopolar cautery. (**c**) View during pituitary gland resection. (**d**) Final view after removal. Legends: [1] sellar dura, [2] pneumatized dorsum sellae, [3] pituitary gland, [4] diaphragma sellae, [5] pituitary stalk retracted by a hook [6] and optic chiasm. Schematic drawing after the figure from Chauvet and Hans [7]

2.3 Summary and Conclusion

Neurosurgery involves a microscopic field with minimal workroom, which creates challenges relating to instrument triangulation and movement. Although neurosurgeons have successfully performed dissections on superficial brain tumors, there are still difficulties in accessing tumors located in deeper areas of the skull. Robotic and robot-assisted endoscopic surgery with its technological advantages could offer a viable solution. Although robotics has been investigated for more than three decades in neurosurgery, clinical applications of robots in neurosurgery are in their infancy. Trans-oral robotic surgery (TORS) has been proposed as a method for accessing the base of the skull, specifically the sella turcica. Reported experience on this subject is limited. TORS has mainly been applied to cadaveric specimens, and there is only one clinical study reporting on four patients with resection of sella turcica tumors resulting in satisfactory outcomes. Therefore, more studies are needed with larger patient sample sizes to confirm TORS as a viable option for accessing the base of the skull.

As by definition the performance of TORS relies on technology, further improvements of medical robots and designing new robotic instruments are necessary steps before TORS can be more widely used by the neurosurgical community.

References

1. Pangal DJ, Cote DJ, Ruzevick J, et al. Robotic and robot-assisted skull base neurosurgery: systematic review of current applications and future directions. Neurosurg Focus. 2022;52(1):E15. https://doi.org/10.3171/2021.10.FOCUS21505.
2. Doulgeris JJ, Gonzalez-Blohm SA, Filis AK, Shea TM, Aghayev K, Vrionis FD. Robotics in neurosurgery: evolution, current challenges, and compromises. Cancer Control. 2015;22(3):352–9. https://doi.org/10.1177/107327481502200314.
3. Carrau RL, Prevedello DM, de Lara D, Durmus K, Ozer E. Combined transoral robotic surgery and endoscopic endonasal approach for the resection of extensive malignancies of the skull base. Head Neck. 2013;35(11):E351–8. https://doi.org/10.1002/hed.23238.
4. Fernandez-Nogueras FJJ, Katati MJ, Arraez Sanchez MA, Molina Martinez M, Sanchez CM. Transoral robotic surgery of the central skull base: preclinical investigations. Eur Arch Otorhinolaryngol. 2014;271(6):1759–63. https://doi.org/10.1007/s00405-013-2717-4.
5. Chauvet D, Missistrano A, Hivelin M, Carpentier A, Cornu P, Hans S. Transoral robotic-assisted skull base surgery to approach the Sella turcica: cadaveric study. Neurosurg Rev. 2014;37(4):609–17. https://doi.org/10.1007/s10143-014-0553-7.
6. Chauvet D, Hans S, Missistrano A, Rebours C, Bakkouri WE, Lot G. Transoral robotic surgery for sellar tumors: first clinical study. J Neurosurg. 2016;127(4):941–8. https://doi.org/10.3171/2016.9.JNS161638.
7. Chauvet D, Hans S. Transoral robotic surgery applied to the skull base. In: Assaad F, Wassmann H, Khodor M, editors. Pituitary diseases. IntechOpen; 2019. https://doi.org/10.5772/intechopen.72984.

3 Robotic Endoscopic Transnasal Skull Base Surgery in Clinical Practice: A Systematic Literature Review

Alba Madoglio, Davide Mattavelli, Marco Ferrari, Elena Roca, Pasquale De Bonis, Marco Maria Fontanella, and Francesco Doglietto

3.1 Introduction

Endoscopic transsphenoidal surgery has recently evolved into endoscopic transnasal skull base surgery (ESBS), which has revolutionized the surgical treatment of sellar and parasellar pathologies [1, 2]. Surgical indications for this approach, which

A. Madoglio · P. De Bonis
Department of Morphology, Surgery and Experimental Medicine, University of Ferrara, Ferrara, Italy

Department of Neurosurgery, Sant' Anna University Hospital, Ferrara, Italy

D. Mattavelli
Unit of Otorhinolaryngology-Head and Neck Surgery, Department of Medical and Surgical Specialties, Radiological Sciences, and Public Health, ASST Spedali Civili of Brescia, University of Brescia, Brescia, Italy

M. Ferrari
Section of Otorhinolaryngology - Head and Neck Surgery, Department of Neurosciences, University of Padua – "Azienda Ospedaliera di Padova", Padua, Italy

E. Roca
Istituto Ospedaliero Fondazione Poliambulanza, Head and Neck Department, Neurosurgery, Brescia, Italy

M. M. Fontanella
Neurosurgery Unit, Department of Medical and Surgical Specialties, Radiological Sciences and Public Health, University of Brescia, Brescia, Italy

F. Doglietto (✉)
Neurosurgery, Department of Neurosciences, Organs and Thorax, Catholic University School of Medicine, Rome, Italy

Neurosurgery, Department of Neuroscience, Fondazione Policlinico Universitario A. Gemelli IRCCS, Rome, Italy
e-mail: francesco.doglietto@unicatt.it

M. M. Al-Salihi et al. (eds.), *Robotics in Skull-Base Surgery*, https://doi.org/10.1007/978-3-031-38376-2_3

takes advantage of the natural corridor provided by the two nostrils and nasal cavities, have expanded thanks to the so-called "extended" approaches, which are usually used to treat complex, even transdural, pathologies. As a consequence, the need for bimanual dissection became evident, and the so-called "two nostrils - four hands technique" was developed [3]. The increasing complexity of ESBS has also led to a significant increase in operating times: physiological tremors and the difficulty of coordinating the movement of the endoscope with surgical instruments in a narrow working space might then become an issue. To address this problem, some teams have suggested the use of a robotic endoscope holder, which should reduce the fatigue of the surgical team and provide both a steady vision and precise micro-movements to optimize the view [4–9].

The use of robotic systems indeed offers a potential solution [8], but the use of robotics in neurosurgery has seen a slower implementation as compared to other specialties [1, 10].

Different prototypes have been described for ESBS [9, 11, 12], but only recently preliminary clinical evaluations have been reported [13–15].

This chapter is a systematic review of the literature to provide a comprehensive critical overview of robotic systems that have been developed for ESBS and evaluated in a clinical setting.

3.2 Material and Methods

A systematic review of papers was performed on PubMed and Scopus using the following search terms and strings to retrieve papers published until August 2022:

- "transnasal AND robotic AND skull base surgery"
- "holder AND robotics AND skull base"
- "endoscopic endonasal AND robot AND pituitary surgery"
- "transsphenoidal AND robotics AND endoscopic AND skull base"
- "clinical evaluation AND robotics AND skull base AND transnasal".

The systematic review is reported according to the PRISMA guidelines [16].

3.2.1 Inclusion and Exclusion Criteria

Studies were included if they reported a clinical evaluation of the robotic system in ESBS and were published in English.

Records were excluded if they were review articles with no novel information or if they reported exclusively preclinical data.

Articles were imported into the reference management software Zotero (Corporation for Digital Scholarship, Roy Rosenzweig Center for History and New Media, George Mason University; Version 6.0.93) and duplicates were removed.

Titles and abstracts of selected records were examined by A.M. and non-relevant citations were excluded.

For each study, the following information was extracted: (1) authors and year of publication, (2) name of the robotic system, (3) function of the robotic system, (4) number of enrolled patients, and (5) key findings.

3.3 Results

A total of 66 studies were identified after the initial search and removal of duplicates. After a review of the abstracts and titles, 10 were selected for full-text analysis. Of these, five articles were included in this systematic literature analysis [13–15, 17, 18]. Articles were excluded for the following reasons: review article (n = 2), preclinical evaluation, or technical descriptions only (*n* = 3). Figure 3.1 shows the flow chart according to the PRISMA statement.

Clinical studies included in the review were divided into the following categories: transoral robotic skull base surgery + ESBS, robotic armrest, and robotic endoscope holders.

The results of this systematic review are summarized in Table 3.1.

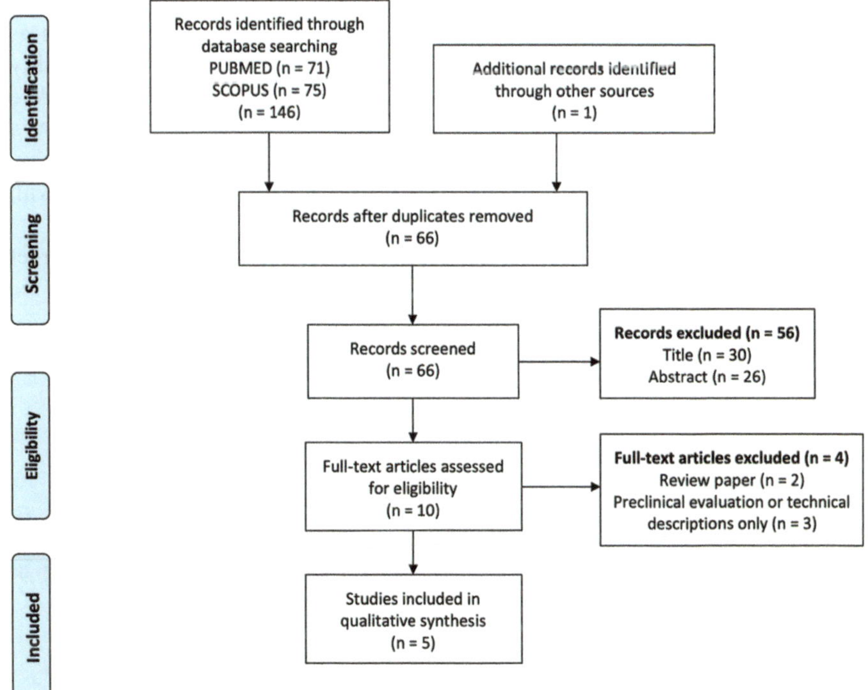

Fig. 3.1 Flow chart according to the PRISMA statement

Table 3.1 Clinical applications of robotic systems in endoscopic skull base surgery: Summary of the results of the systematic literature review, reporting the robotic systems that have been applied to endoscopic skull base surgery (see text for further details)

First Author (year of publication)	Robotic System	Function	Approach	No. of patients enrolled	Intraoperative complications	Key findings
Carrau et al. (2013) [18]	da Vinci (intuitive surgical; Sunnyvale, CA)	–	Transoral / endoscopic endonasal	2	No complications related to the use of this system	– TORS approach for inferior aspects and EEA for superior aspects of tumor resulted in favorable operative outcomes – EEA-TORS combined technique evades many of the morbidities related to open approaches (i.e., issues related to skin incision, need for bony osteotomies, and risk of osteonecrosis)
Ogiwara et al. (2017) [17]	iArms (DENSO Corp.)	Armrest	Endonasal / Transsphenoidal	43	No complications related to the use of this system	– Three modes: Transfer (free), arm holding (hold), and arm free (wait) – Reduced fatigue, hand trembling, and improved surgeon comfort
Hintschich et al. (2021) [13]	ENDOFIX exo (AKTORmed, barbing, Germany)	Endoscope holder	Endonasal / Transsphenoidal / Prelacrimal-transmaxillar / combined endonasal and external /Transoral	30	No complications related to the use of this system	– Electromagnetic manual support arm to hold the endoscope with six DoF – Fixed clamp, easy to sterilize, and low cost
Mattheis et al. (2021) [15]	Endoscope robot® (Medineering, Munich, Germany)	Endoscope holder	A combined approach transnasally and laterally via a small skin incision (orbital decompression)	8	No adverse events or complications	– Endoscopic orbital surgery – Safe and effective endoscope support
Zappa et al. (2021) [14]	Endoscope robot® (Medineering, Munich, Germany)	Endoscope holder	Endonasal / Transsphenoidal	21	No complications related to the use of this system	– Objective advantages for visualization – Subjective benefits for “complex” scenarios – Subjective limits for first positioning

3.3.1 Transoral Robotic Surgery (TORS) Combined with an Extended Endonasal Approach (EEA-TORS)

Carrau et al. [18] described the use of a combined TORS approach and ESBS, which was studied on anatomical specimens, and then applied clinically to two patients (Table 3.1).

In the first clinical case, an MRI of the neck and skull base revealed an infiltrating tumor with probable origin in the nasopharynx and extending to the sphenoid sinus, clivus, middle cranial fossa, and infratemporal fossa with striking perineural involvement of V3. A transpterygoid EEA with surgical navigation assistance exposed the tumor adequately except for that part that extended below the level of the hard palate, which was addressed with TORS using the da Vinci surgical system.

The second patient presented an extensive tumor, compatible with a chordoma, involving the posterior and middle cranial base that extended to the cranial cervical junction and down to C1/C2. Endonasal approach was useful for exposure of the tumor down to C1, while a transoral approach was chosen to remove the tumor extending to C2.

The Authors concluded that TORS and ESBS are complementary techniques that, when combined, provide excellent exposure to the posterior skull base, nasopharynx, and infratemporal fossa. The main advantage of TORS for managing skull base tumors is the ability to reach the posterior skull base below the level of the Eustachian tube, which is the inferior limit of the EEA. This study confirms the current limits of robotics, as the ESBS phase was not performed with the robot [5].

3.3.2 Robotic Armrest

Ogiwara et al. [17] described the iArms (DENSO Corp.), a robotic armrest that allows neurosurgeons to rest their non-dominant arm, which holds the endoscope, thus reducing fatigue and increasing stability. The system has three modes: transfer (Free), arms holding (Hold), and arm free (Wait). When the surgeon's arm is placed on the arm holder, the mode changes from Wait to Hold. When the surgeon's arm moves to the desired position and holds still, the mode changes from Free to Hold. The mode is changed from Hold to Free with a click action by the surgeon's arm.

The authors reported on the application of this robotic device to endoscopic endonasal transsphenoidal surgery and evaluated their initial clinical experience with 43 patients with different pathologies (i.e., 29 with pituitary adenoma, 3 with meningioma, 3 with Rathke's cleft cyst, 2 with craniopharyngioma, 2 with chordoma, and 4 with other conditions). The intelligent armrest proved to be safe and effective. The main limit of the system is that it does not substitute the surgeon's arm but is indeed an armrest [5, 8].

3.3.3 Robotic Endoscope Holders

The ENDOFIXexo system [8] (AKTORmed) is a robotic endoscope holder, originally used for abdominal procedures and then successfully modified for sinus surgery. Hintschich et al. [13] reported its use in a clinical trial of 30 patients, of whom 11 underwent transsphenoidal resection of a pituitary adenoma. This holder is an electromagnetic manual support arm to hold the endoscope and it has six different degrees of freedom (DoF). It combines three fundamental requirements of an endoscope holding arm: intuitive maneuverability, flexibility, and high stability; thus, the surgeon can operate in a bimanual action. However, in transnasal surgery, the accessibility is restricted to the posterior ethmoid and the sphenoid sinus or dependent on the partial resection of the nasal septum. With a bimanual action, endoscopic surgery may not be limited to paranasal sinuses and the frontal skull base, but expand to other operating sites.

Recently, Zappa et al. [14, 19] described a hybrid robotic solution for ESBS in a preclinical [19] and clinical [14] setting (*Endoscope Robot*®, Medineering, Munich, Germany). It is a compact robot that was specifically developed to work as an endoscope holder during transnasal interventions and is made of a robotic arm coupled with a smaller robot that acts as an endoscope holder. The positioning arm has seven DoF: it can be driven in every position of space by the simultaneous manual unlocking of two joints (Fig. 3.2). Its distal end is connected to the endoscope holder. Once attached to the holder and positioned inside the nasal cavity, the endoscope can be oriented upward, downward, or laterally using the joystick of a foot pedal (Fig. 3.2). Furthermore, it can be moved in or out by pressing different pads on the foot pedal. Also, a specific button has the function of making the robot return to a previously saved "home position" at any moment during surgery.

Zappa et al. provided a preclinical evaluation of the potential advantages and surgeons' first impressions of a hybrid robotic solution for ESBS. Endoscope Robot® seems to provide a benefit to the single surgeon with experience in bimanual endoscopic surgery [19]. The Brescia group then described the first clinical series of robotic endoscopic transnasal surgery, providing a clinical evaluation of the potential advantages of this novel hybrid solution and the surgeons' subjective impressions (Table 3.1). Twenty-one patients underwent robot-assisted endoscopic transsphenoidal surgery for different pathologies (i.e., 16 pituitary adenomas, 3 chordomas, 1 craniopharyngioma, and 1 pituitary exploration for Cushing's disease) for a total of 23 procedures (one patient underwent two endoscopic revisions of a skull base reconstruction) [14].

When compared to a matched, historical cohort of patients, clinical results were comparable. Video analyses of the two cohorts (hand-held endoscopy vs. robotic) documented significant differences in endoscope lens cleaning and position readjustments, as they were significantly less frequent in the robotic procedures. Subjective advantages reported by surgeons included smoothness of movement, image steadiness, and improvement of maneuvers in narrow spaces and with angled endoscopes.

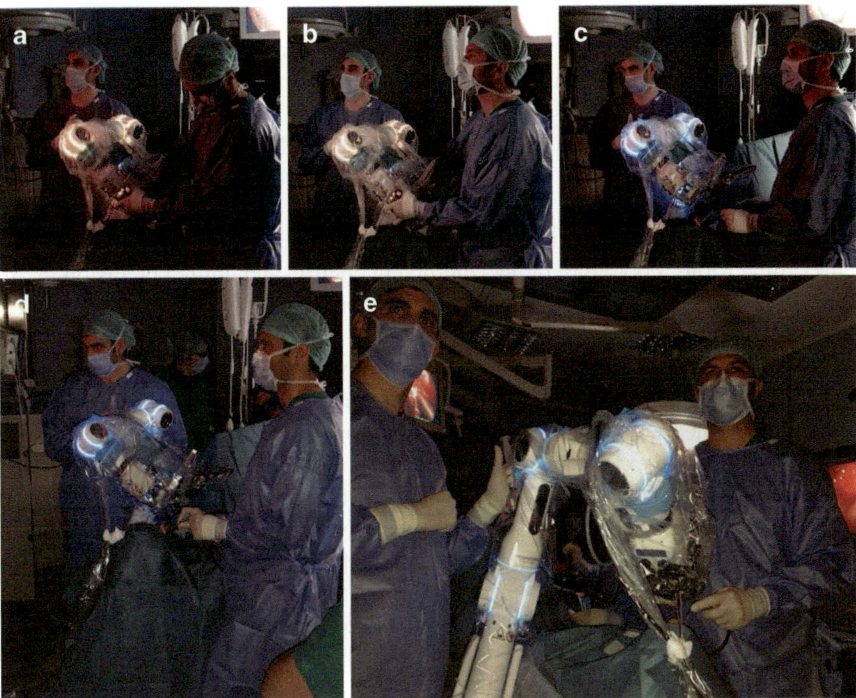

Fig. 3.2 Clinical evaluation at the University of Brescia. (**a**–**c**) Sequence (from a 5-seconds video) of Endoscope Robot® positioning in the operating room for endoscopic transnasal skull base surgery. The system is unlocked, and the surgeon manually positions the robotic endoscope holder (**a**, **b**) in the nose; this is usually performed after the nasal corridor has been created. The system is then locked and ready for use (**c**). (**d**, **e**) Surgeons' positions during the robotic phase (i.e., bimanual and during tumor removal) of endoscopic transnasal skull base surgery: the endoscope is held by the robot, which is controlled by a foot pedal (see text for further details)

The present limits of the system were also highlighted: intraoperative endonasal positioning always took less than 8 min, but was the less valued robotic phase due to the perceived weight of the system when the robotic holder had to be fully unblocked for significant changes in the endoscope position (i.e., from outside the surgical field to the intranasal corridor—Fig. 3.2). Furthermore, an ergonomic limit became evident, as the primary surgeon's weight is predominantly on the right foot during the robotic phase, as the left is used to control the movements of the robot.

The same robotic system was recently applied to endoscopic orbital surgery by Mattheis et al. who reported the results of orbital decompression with Medineering Robotic Endoscope Guiding System [15]. The system, though, is no longer commercially available.

3.4 Discussion

The aim of this review was to depict the clinical use of robotic systems in ESBS and identify the potential benefits and limitations for future optimizations.

Despite different preclinical studies have been published, this review confirms that, clinical experience on robotic ESBS is sparse and scattered on different robotic models.

Prototypes described in preclinical evaluation have some limitations, including bulky dimensions, poor ergonomics, inefficient control, and limited precision [4, 5]; this aspect probably explains why most of them have not been tested in clinical practice yet.

Only two robotic endoscope holders have been described in clinical studies [13–15], while others reported the use of a robotic arm rest [17] or transoral robotic surgery combined with an extended endonasal approach [18].

The very limited experience with the da Vinci system (only 2 cases in 2013, and none published thereafter) witness the difficulty to adapt to ESBS robotic systems that were conceived for different clinical scenarios.

The most promising prototypes are those helping the holding of the endoscope (armrest or endoscopic holder), allowing for an easier bimanual dissection.

The benefits of those robotic systems included reduced operator fatigue, especially in case of lengthy bimanual procedures, in small working spaces; stability of endoscopic image; absence of misunderstood verbal commands between the surgeon and assistant since the robot can be controlled directly by the primary surgeon [8, 14].

Endoscope Robot® is apparently the best option so far, since it can guarantee a wider degree of maneuverability (with robotic-controlled micro-movements for fine adjustments) to optimize visualization during any phase of dissection. Besides the previously cited advantages, one of the most relevant benefits perceived with this system is the robotic maneuvering of angled endoscopes or any endoscopes close to the target and in narrow spaces [14]. Despite the potential benefits, Zappa et al. [14] also underlined the present limits of the system: the main one is the perception of the weight of the system at the first positioning inside the surgical corridor. Near future developments are expected to address this limitation, as the arm that holds the small robotic holder is robotic as well.

Another possible drawback of the application of robotic systems to ESBS is the need to design and develop dedicated models for this kind of surgery, which is rare and performed in a few, highly specialized centers. As a consequence, the commercial interest of the companies to invest in these solutions may represent a limiting factor. Overall, we believe that the robotic phase of ESBS is just at its dawn: the current hybrid solutions have already shown benefits even in the clinical setting. The need for close collaboration with the industry and engineering research centers is evident and of paramount importance for future developments.

3.5 Conclusion

A few clinical applications of robotic endoscopic skull base surgery have been described. To improve the present results, a true multidisciplinary collaboration is required, with novel solutions in terms of robot control to fully exploit the advantages of robotic holders for endoscopic skull base surgery.

Disclosure The Authors declare no Conflict of Interest.

References

1. Cote DJ, Ruzevick J, Strickland BA, Zada G. Commentary: hybrid robotics for endoscopic Transnasal Skull Base surgery: single-Centre case series. Oper Neurosurg. 2021;21(6):E471
2. Doglietto F, Prevedello DM, Jane JA, Han J, Laws ER. A brief history of endoscopic transsphenoidal surgery—from Philipp Bozzini to the first world congress of endoscopic Skull Base surgery. Neurosurg Focus. 2005;19(6):1–6.
3. Castelnuovo P, Pistochini A, Locatelli D. Different surgical approaches to the sellar region: focusing on the "two nostrils four hands technique." Rhinology 2006 44(1):2–7.
4. Bolzoni Villaret A, Doglietto F, Carobbio A, Schreiber A, Panni C, Piantoni E, et al. Robotic Transnasal endoscopic Skull Base surgery: systematic review of the literature and report of a novel prototype for a hybrid system (Brescia endoscope assistant robotic holder). World Neurosurg. 2017;105:875–83.
5. Madoglio A, Zappa F, Mattavelli D, Rampinelli V, Ferrari M, Schreiber A, et al. Robotics in endoscopic transnasal skull base surgery: Literature review and personal experience. In: Control systems design of bio-robotics and bio-mechatronics with advanced applications [Internet]. Elsevier; 2020 [cited 2021 Feb 7]. p. 221–244. Available from: https://linkinghub.elsevier.com/retrieve/pii/B9780128174630000083
6. Chan JYK, Leung I, Navarro-Alarcon D, Lin W, Li P, Lee DLY, et al. Foot-controlled robotic-enabled endoscope holder for endoscopic sinus surgery: a cadaveric feasibility study. Laryngoscope. 2016;126(3):566–9.
7. Blanco RGF, Boahene K. Robotic-assisted skull base surgery: preclinical study. J Laparoendosc Adv Surg Tech A. 2013;23(9):776–82.
8. Pangal DJ, Cote DJ, Ruzevick J, Yarovinsky B, Kugener G, Wrobel B, et al. Robotic and robot-assisted skull base neurosurgery: systematic review of current applications and future directions. Neurosurg Focus. 2022;52(1):E15.
9. Nimsky C, Rachinger J, Iro H, Fahlbusch R. Adaptation of a hexapod-based robotic system for extended endoscope-assisted transsphenoidal skull base surgery. Minim Invasive Neurosurg MIN. 2004;47(1):41–6.
10. Madoglio A, Roca E, Tampalini F, Fontanella MM, Doglietto F. Robotics in Neuroendoscopy. In: Al-Salihi MM, Tubbs RS, Ayyad A, Goto T, Maarouf M, editors. Introduction to robotics in minimally invasive neurosurgery [internet]. Cham: Springer International Publishing; 2022[cited 2022 Aug 21]. p. 39–55. Available from: https://doi.org/10.1007/978-3-030-90862-1_4.
11. Wurm J, Dannenmann T, Bohr C, Iro H, Bumm K. Increased safety in robotic paranasal sinus and skull base surgery with redundant navigation and automated registration. Int J Med Robot. 2005;1(3):42–8.
12. Wei X, Zhang Y, Ju F, Guo H, Chen B, Wu H. Design and analysis of a continuum robot for transnasal skull base surgery. Int J Med Robot [Internet]. 2021 Dec [cited 2022 Aug 15];17(6). Available from: https://onlinelibrary.wiley.com/doi/10.1002/rcs.2328

13. Hintschich CA, Fischer R, Seebauer C, Schebesch KM, Bohr C, Kühnel T. A third hand to the surgeon: the use of an endoscope holding arm in endonasal sinus surgery and well beyond. Eur Arch Otorhinolaryngol. 2022;279(4):1891–8.
14. Zappa F, Madoglio A, Ferrari M, Mattavelli D, Schreiber A, Taboni S, et al. Hybrid robotics for endoscopic Transnasal Skull Base surgery: single-Centre case series. Oper Neurosurg. 2021;21(6):426–35.
15. Mattheis S, Schlüter A, Stähr K, Holtmann L, Höing B, Hussain T, et al. First use of a new robotic endoscope guiding system in endoscopic orbital decompression. Ear Nose Throat J. 2021;100(5_suppl):443S–8S.
16. Moher D, Liberati A, Tetzlaff J, Altman DG, for the PRISMA Group. Preferred reporting items for systematic reviews and meta-analyses: the PRISMA statement. BMJ. 2009;339(jul21 1):b2535.
17. Ogiwara T, Goto T, Nagm A, Hongo K. Endoscopic endonasal transsphenoidal surgery using the iArmS operation support robot: initial experience in 43 patients. Neurosurg Focus. 2017;42(5):E10.
18. Carrau RL, Prevedello DM, de Lara D, Durmus K, Ozer E. Combined transoral robotic surgery and endoscopic endonasal approach for the resection of extensive malignancies of the skull base: combined TORS and EEA for resection of extensive malignancies of Skull Base. Head Neck. 2013;35(11):E351–8.
19. Zappa F, Mattavelli D, Madoglio A, Rampinelli V, Ferrari M, Tampalini F, et al. Hybrid robotics for endoscopic Skull Base surgery: preclinical evaluation and surgeon first impression. World Neurosurg. 2020;134:e572–80.

4 Robotics in Sinus Surgery

Alexandros Andrianakis and Peter Valentin Tomazic

4.1 Introduction

In contrast to head and neck surgery or even skull base surgery, robotics in sinus surgery has been limited thus far [1]. The only approved system is the da Vinci robot, which has been successfully implemented in, e.g., thyroid surgery or surgery for oropharyngeal or hypopharyngeal cancers [1]. The biggest challenges are the size of the instruments/robotic arms and the port, which is limited by the nostrils. Another big limitation is that transnasal endoscopic instruments are traditionally rigid, and flexible instruments are required for optimal benefits of robotic surgery, costing space.

4.2 Robotic Endoscope Holders

For those reasons, robotic endoscope holders have received most attention in endoscopic sinus surgery. The advantage of these holders is that the surgeon has both hands free to manipulate instruments. Eichhorn et al. [2] published a trial with 16 procedures with and without robot-assisted guidance and found a learning curve, especially regarding the duration of surgeries. One problem with endoscope holders is their maneuverability, since it is desirable for surgeons to be able to keep their hands free for the instruments, not to steer the scope. Chan et al. [3, 4] designed a Foot-controlled Robot-Enabled EnDOscope Manipulator (FREEDOM) for this purpose. Here, the surgeon has a Bluetooth device fixed on his foot and can guide the robot arm by moving the foot, keeping both hands free. Since the device is braced on the foot, movement in all space directions is granted. This is a clear advantage

A. Andrianakis · P. V. Tomazic (✉)
Department of General ORL, H&NS, Medical University of Graz, Graz, Austria
e-mail: peter.tomazic@medunigraz.at

M. M. Al-Salihi et al. (eds.), *Robotics in Skull-Base Surgery*,
https://doi.org/10.1007/978-3-031-38376-2_4

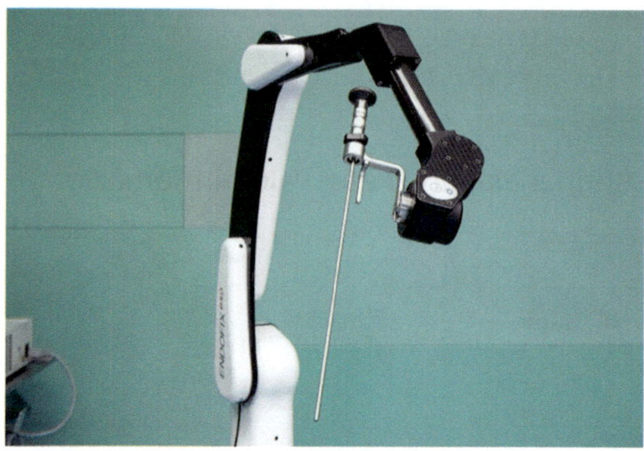

Fig. 4.1 The three electromagnetic locks of the ENDOFIXexo allow any position to be taken within arm range. Reference: Hintschich, C. A., Fischer, R., Seebauer, C., Schebesch, K.-M., Bohr, C. & Kühnel, T. (2021). A third hand to the surgeon: the use of an endoscope holding arm in endonasal sinus surgery and well beyond. *European Archives of Oto-Rhino-Laryngology*, *279*(4), 1891–1898. https://doi.org/10.1007/s00405-021-06935-x

over other systems such as ENDOFIXexo (Fig. 4.1), which is oriented with a control button similar to moving microscopes [5]. Friedrich et al. [6] described a similar robotic arm system with four segments and seven degrees of freedom operated by a foot pedal and a joystick. They published the feasibility of this system on a cadaveric head inclusive of implementing the EndoCAMeleon endoscope, which allows vision angulation to be adjusted freely by a steering wheel on the endoscope shaft (without steps). This is an additional advantage of not having to change endoscopes at the robot arm when angled vision (e.g., frontal sinus) is required.

Another interesting aspect of robotic arm-assisted sinus surgery was explored by Okuda et al. [7]. They investigated the time needed for lens-wiping during surgery, comparing the so-called iArmS Robotic system to standard endoscopy. Since the endpoints were blinded in advance, the surgeons could not know the aim of the study. The surgeries were recorded and intervals for lens-wiping were measured; there was a highly significant prolongation when the iArmS system was used. Here, an automated lens cleaning/flushing system could help; however, this has not yet been investigated. Given the necessity of operating such systems by a foot pedal, it would give the surgeon an additional tool on top of maneuvering the robotic arms.

4.3 Steerable Flexible Endoscopes

Another innovation, especially for maxillary sinus surgery, is steerable flexible endoscopes. Most instruments described share the problem of size; their large diameters would not allow insertion to be atraumatic unless wider resections and antrostomies were performed. Legrand et al. published a feasibility study on the so-called PliENT flexible endoscope (Fig. 4.2) for maxillary sinus surgery [8]. This

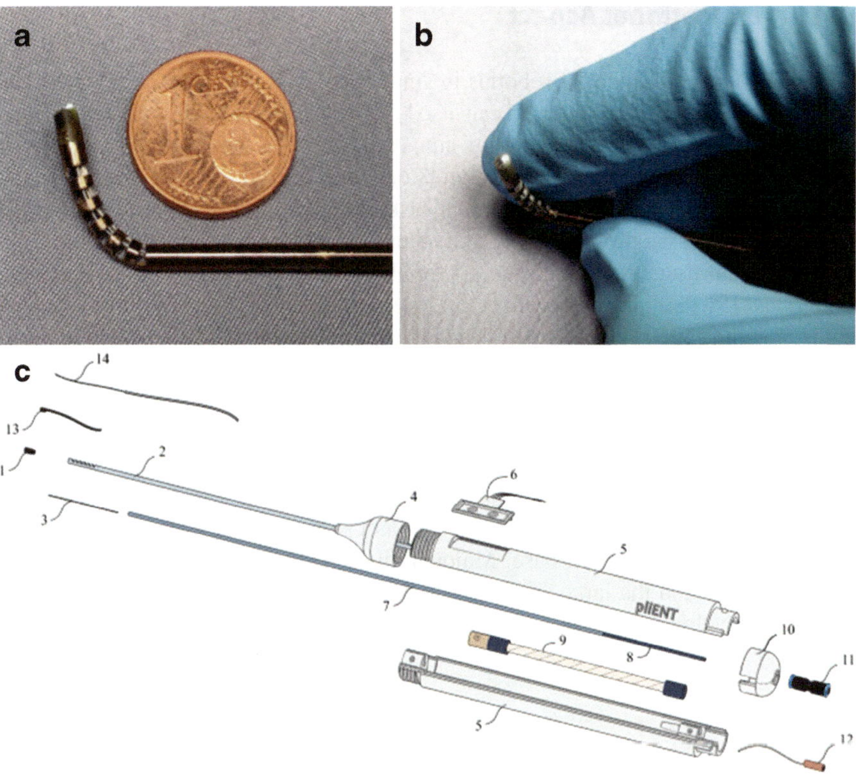

Fig. 4.2 Flexible endoscope for maxillary sinus inspection. (**a**) View of the bending capabilities of the 2.3-mm diameter endoscope; (**b**) detail of the endoscope distal tip with camera and illumination; (**c**) overview of the different components of the single-handed, flexible, steerable endoscope for maxillary sinus surgery. (1) Tip; (2) NiTi shaft; (3) cable; (4) screw-on cap; (5) two-parts handle; (6) button interface; (7) mobile outer tube of the concentric muscle; (8) fixed inner tube of the concentric muscle; (9) McKibben muscle; (10) plug-on cap; (11) pressure source connector; (12) pressure source tube; (13) chip-on-tip camera; (14). light fiber. Reference: Legrand, J., Ourak, M., Gerven, L. V., Poorten, V. V., Poorten, E. V. (2022). A miniature robotic steerable endoscope for maxillary sinus surgery called PliENT. Scientific Reports, 12(1), 2299. 10.1038/s41598-022-05969-3

endoscope is steerable with two buttons and can be inserted into the maxillary sinus without wide antrostomies. Compared to standard endoscopes, the PliENT could provide a wide view of the posterior and lateral walls only by antrostomies, and partial views (>50%) of the medial wall, the floor, and the anterior wall. For standard scopes, this was only possible for types 3 and 4 maxillectomies, respectively, in 0° and 30° lenses. The scope is a single-use design, but it meets the criteria for sterilization.

4.4 Educational Aspect

Another important aspect of robotics in sinus surgery is training. Cadaveric specimens are not always available and can also be costly. Animal models are feasible but do not always reflect the anatomy of human sinuses. To overcome problems with training on cadaver heads, various simulators have been proposed. With a virtual-based haptic system, different surgical tasks could be accomplished, giving the trainee the impression of operating in a natural environment. Here, the haptic feedback can train tissue resistance and potentially give feedback about risks and complications [9]. Future perspectives in training definitely lie in virtual reality environments and 3D printing systems that can simulate real tissues from mucosa to bone optimally [10, 11].

4.5 Conclusion and Future Perspective

At present, the robotic systems available are not suited to endoscopic surgery of the paranasal sinuses and skull base. Major limitations include the lack of a drilling/suction device and the large size of the instruments/robotic arms. With continuing technical developments, the potential of robots for endoscopic sinus surgery will definitely increase in the future.

References

1. Schneider JS, Burgner J, Webster RJ, Russell PT. Robotic surgery for the sinuses and skull base: what are the possibilities and what are the obstacles? Curr Opin Otolaryngol Head Neck Surg. 2013;21(1):11–6. https://doi.org/10.1097/moo.0b013e32835bc650.
2. Eichhorn KW, Westphal R, Rilk M, Last C, Bootz F, Wahl F, Jakob M, Send T. Robot-assisted endoscope guidance versus manual endoscope guidance in functional endonasal sinus surgery (FESS). Acta Otolaryngol. 2017;137(10):1090–5. https://doi.org/10.1080/00016489.2017.1336284.
3. Chan JYK, Leung I, Navarro-Alarcon D, Lin W, Li P, Lee DLY, Liu Y, Tong MCF. Foot-controlled robotic-enabled endoscope holder for endoscopic sinus surgery: a cadaveric feasibility study. Laryngoscope. 2015;126(3):566–9. https://doi.org/10.1002/lary.25634.
4. Zhong F, Li P, Shi J, Wang Z, Wu J, Chan JYK, Leung N, Leung I, Tong MCF, Liu Y-H. Foot-controlled robot-enabled EnDOscope manipulator (FREEDOM) for sinus surgery: design, control, and evaluation. IEEE Trans Biomed Eng. 2019;67(6):1530–41. https://doi.org/10.1109/tbme.2019.2939557.
5. Hintschich CA, Fischer R, Seebauer C, Schebesch K-M, Bohr C, Kühnel T. A third hand to the surgeon: the use of an endoscope holding arm in endonasal sinus surgery and well beyond. Eur Arch Otorhinolaryngol. 2021;279(4):1891–8. https://doi.org/10.1007/s00405-021-06935-x.
6. Friedrich D, Sommer F, Scheithauer M, Greve J, Hoffmann T, Schuler P. An innovate robotic endoscope guidance system for Transnasal sinus and Skull Base surgery: proof of concept. J Neurol Surg Part B Skull Base. 2017;78(06):466–72. https://doi.org/10.1055/s-0037-1603974.
7. Okuda H, Okamoto J, Takumi Y, Kakehata S, Muragaki Y. The iArmS Robotic Armrest Prolongs Endoscope Lens–Wiping Intervals in Endoscopic Sinus Surgery. Surg Innov. 2020;27(5):515–22. https://doi.org/10.1177/1553350620929864.

8. Legrand J, Ourak M, Gerven LV, Poorten VV, Poorten EV. A miniature robotic steerable endoscope for maxillary sinus surgery called PliENT. Sci Rep. 2022;12(1):2299. https://doi.org/10.1038/s41598-022-05969-3.
9. Sadeghnejad S, Khadivar F, Abdollahi E, Moradi H, Farahmand F, Hosseini SMS, Vossoughi G. A validation study of a virtual-based haptic system for endoscopic sinus surgery training. Int J Med Robotics + Comp Assist Surg MRCAS. 2019;15(6):e2039. https://doi.org/10.1002/rcs.2039.
10. Alrasheed AS, Nguyen LHP, Mongeau L, Funnell WRJ, Tewfik MA. Development and validation of a 3D-printed model of the ostiomeatal complex and frontal sinus for endoscopic sinus surgery training: 3D-printed endoscopic sinus surgery simulator. Int Forum Allergy Rhinol. 2017;7(8):837–41. https://doi.org/10.1002/alr.21960.
11. Varshney R, Frenkiel S, Nguyen LHP, Young M, Maestro RD, Zeitouni A, Tewfik MA, Canada NRC. Development of the McGill simulator for endoscopic sinus surgery: a new high-fidelity virtual reality simulator for endoscopic sinus surgery. Am J Rhinol Allergy. 2014;28(4):330–4.

5 Robotics for Approaches to the Anterior Cranial Fossa

Miracle C. Anokwute, Alexei Christodoulides,
Raewyn G. Campbell, Richard J. Harvey,
and Antonio Di Ieva

5.1 Historical and Current Methods in Anterior Cranial Fossa Approaches

Depending on the pathology within the anterior cranial fossa, classic surgical approaches can be classified into two broad categories: open, versus minimal access or minimally invasive. Historically, open approaches, usually relying on access via midfacial approaches, bicoronal craniotomies for subfrontal or interhemispheric approaches, pterional, or orbitozygomatic, were often employed to access structures within the anterior cranial fossa. Pathologies addressed in this way include skull

M. C. Anokwute
Faculty of Medicine, Health and Human Sciences, Macquarie Medical School, Macquarie University, Sydney, NSW, Australia

Department of Neurosurgery, Indiana University School of Medicine, Indianapolis, IN, USA

A. Christodoulides
Department of Neurosurgery, Indiana University School of Medicine, Indianapolis, IN, USA

R. G. Campbell
Faculty of Medicine, Health and Human Sciences, Macquarie Medical School, Macquarie University, Sydney, NSW, Australia

R. J. Harvey
Faculty of Medicine, Health and Human Sciences, Macquarie Medical School, Macquarie University, Sydney, NSW, Australia

Rhinology and Skull Base Research Group, Applied Medical Research Centre, University of New South Wales, Sydney, NSW, Australia

A. Di Ieva (✉)
Faculty of Medicine, Health and Human Sciences, Macquarie Medical School, Macquarie University, Sydney, NSW, Australia

Computational NeuroSurgery (CNS) Lab, Macquarie University, Sydney, NSW, Australia
e-mail: antonio.diieva@mq.edu.au

M. M. Al-Salihi et al. (eds.), *Robotics in Skull-Base Surgery*,
https://doi.org/10.1007/978-3-031-38376-2_5

base tumors (e.g., meningiomas and sellar tumors) and carcinomas, anterior circle of Willis aneurysms, anterior encephaloceles, and facial, orbital and/or anterior skull base fractures [1–10]. Morales-Valero et al. offered a comprehensive historical overview focusing on the use of craniotomies for anterior cranial fossa meningiomas [11]. Although open approaches are still used in specific cases, minimal access approaches relying on surgical microscopes, endoscopes, and/or exoscopes have grown in popularity during the 50 years since they were introduced.

Minimal access approaches in anterior cranial fossa operations are not new to neurosurgery and skull base surgery; the first transsphenoidal approach to remove a pituitary tumor was performed in 1907 by Dr. Hermann Schloffer via a superior nasal route through a transfacial lateral rhinotomy incision [12]. However, the introduction of the operating microscope to neurosurgery by Dr. Theodore Kurze during the late 1950s meant such minimal access approaches could be undertaken more confidently, so the technique was adopted swiftly [13]. Further improvements to microscope design by neurosurgeons including Dr. Gazi Yaşargil meant greater mobility and ease of visualization during microscopic surgery [13–15].

The first transsphenoidal approach to a pituitary tumor using a microscope was conducted in 1962 by Dr. Jules Hardy [16]. Further adoption/development of techniques such as endonasal endoscopy for anterior skull base surgery made it easier to see inside the tight cavities, as needed for minimally invasive access to the anterior cranial fossa [17]. The value of endonasal endoscopy for resection of pituitary tumors via a transsphenoidal approach was first demonstrated in 1977 [18]. The pure endonasal endoscopic approach to pituitary lesions was first adopted at the Universities of Toronto and Pittsburgh in 1996 while others were using the endoscope as a mere adjunct to the microscope for transnasal procedures [19, 20]. Another minimal access approach to the anterior cranial fossa made possible by the endoscope and/or intraoperative microscope is the endoscopic-assisted supraorbital keyhole approach [21–26]. This has been used for resecting meningiomas within the anterior cranial fossa and for treating aneurysms [22, 27].

Currently, an extended endonasal endoscopic approach for access to the anterior cranial fossa is preferred when feasible. Numerous studies have compared endoscopic and microscopic surgeries for tumor resections in the anterior cranial fossa, and the data suggest that endoscopic surgeries provide superior outcomes such as gross total resection or postoperative meningitis rates in functioning versus non-functioning pituitary adenomas [28–32]. Endoscopic transsphenoidal approaches have also proved superior to transcranial approaches for resecting tuberculum sellae meningiomas even with optic canal invasion [2]. Minimal access techniques for access to the anterior cranial fossa have benefits over craniotomy-based approaches. These include minimal retraction and manipulation of the brain with accompanying neurovascular structures and increased visualization of the surrounding anatomy [33–35]. Although the benefits of endoscopic and microscopic techniques are tremendous, there are many drawbacks. First, numerous studies report the ergonomic difficulties associated with operating tools such as endoscopes and their potential musculoskeletal effects on surgeons [36, 37]. Additionally, the rigidity of endoscopes often makes it difficult to navigate the regional anatomy of the cranium, paranasal sinuses, and nasal cavities with limited 2D fields of view secondary to the limited degrees of freedom of the endoscope [34]. The endoscopic approach also requires a specific training curve in the anatomy laboratory [38, 39]. Surgical instruments used for minimal access approaches are often limited by their rigidity, making tasks such as suturing, hemostasis, and retraction difficult within such confined spaces. Many of the drawbacks associated with both microscopic and endoscopic techniques have to an extent been addressed by the relatively recent development of surgical exoscopes for neurosurgical use [40]. The literature documents a wide spectrum of exoscope uses, ranging from educational purposes in cadaver labs to tumor resection and implantation of vagus nerve stimulators [41–44]. Specific to the anterior cranial fossa, exoscopic approaches have been used to treat dural arteriovenous fistulas, craniopharyngiomas, and pituitary adenomas, and to clip aneurysms, to name just a few pathologies [45–47]. Montemurro et al. comprehensively summarized the current state of exoscope use in both cranial- and spine-based neurosurgery [48]. Continuing advances with exoscopes allowing for improvements in depth-perception and better visualization in narrow surgical corridors will surely allow exoscope use to increase. Needless to say, endoscopic and exoscopic techniques have proved complementary in several scenarios, including anterior and anterolateral skull base craniofacial resections [47].

5.2 Brief Overview of Robotic Skull Base Surgery

Robotic skull base surgery is defined by the surgical robotic type, surgical approach, and anatomical constraints of the trajectory to the lesion. Currently, robotic anterior skull base surgery is in its infancy, with limited applications to patient care. Mostly, it is still being extrapolated from computer modeling and cadaveric approaches to live patients as the robots are being developed to overcome the challenges associated with robotic skull base surgery [49].

Surgical robots for the skull base are classed as passive, semi-active, or active systems. Robots that require the surgeon's input to direct and maneuver them are passive systems. They are also described as surgically assistive robots and include robots that act as instrument holders. Semi-active systems provide robotic guidance to the surgeon, for example, mechanical guidance with drilling. Active system robots function autonomously and carry out surgical tasks independently as they receive information from their environment [50–52].

Active systems are subclassified into supervisor-controlled, tele-surgical, or shared control. In supervisor-controlled systems, the robot automatically performs a surgical task while the surgeon supervises it. Tele-surgical active systems are controlled by the surgeon in real time via haptic feedback. Shared-control active systems give full control to the surgeon as the robot provides steady manipulation of instruments [50–52]. Another broad classification of robotic anterior skull base systems is true surgical robots versus experimental robots; i.e., those ready for patient care versus cadaver laboratory use [50–56].

5.3 Robotic Surgical Approaches to the Anterior Skull Base

The ultimate goals of robotic anterior skull base surgery are to limit brain retraction, provide more direct exposure and access to pathological lesions, decrease neurovascular manipulation, improve visualization, and limit morbidity/mortality while improving patient outcomes [34]. These approaches also provide improved ergonomics for the surgeon, reducing surgeon fatigue and musculoskeletal injuries [34, 57, 58]. Below, we have divided these approaches into single versus multi-portal/combined methods, each category further subdivided on the basis of anatomical approach.

5.3.1 Single Portal

5.3.1.1 Transoral Robotic Surgery

Transoral robotic surgery (TORS) was the initial robotic approach to lesions of the oropharynx and nasopharynx. This was adapted by Lee and colleagues in 2010 for skull base lesions [59] (Fig. 5.1).

They used three arms of the da Vinci Surgical System Robot (Intuitive Surgical; Sunnyvale, California, USA) for TORS skull base approaches on seven cadavers. The cadaver heads were positioned supine with a Crowe-Davis retractor (Storz; Heidelberg, Germany) inserted into the oral cavity [59]. The approach required retraction of the soft palate after two rubber catheters were inserted through the nose, brought out laterally through the mouth and then clamped in position. With the da Vinci robot (Intuitive Surgical; Sunnyvale, California, USA) at the head of the table, its three arms were angled and placed in the mouth while avoiding buccal compression. One arm held either an 8.5-mm diameter 0° or 30° angled endoscope placed through the mouth in the midline. The other two arms held 5 mm diameter articulating EndoWrist instruments placed transorally. A midline incision along the

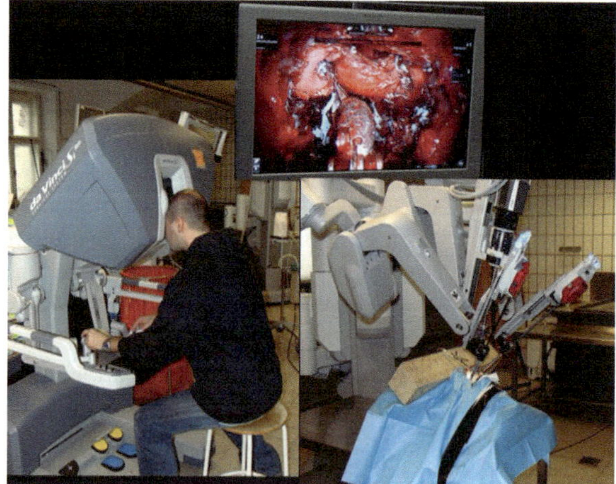

Fig. 5.1 Author Antonio Di Ieva's anatomy demonstration of using the da Vinci robot for a transoral approach to the anterior and middle skull base (Centre for Anatomy and Cell Biology, Department of Systematic Anatomy, Medical University of Vienna, Vienna, Austria, 2011)

posterior pharyngeal mucosa was made by the surgeon controlling the robot from the console. The assistant surgeon stood beside the head to assist and monitor clearance of the robotic arms. The clivus, foramen magnum, and eustachian tubes were identified. Once the bone was identified following soft tissue dissection, the assistant surgeon used a matchstick burr (AM-8) for drilling. After the clivus was identified, a sphenoidectomy was performed. The 30° endoscope was angled cephalad to allow the sella, tuberculum sellae, and planum sphenoidale to be visualized. However, the robotic arms were at their maximum extension at this point and could not angle more cephalad owing to the restrictions of the oral aperture [53, 59]. Despite this disadvantage, Chauvet and colleagues successfully performed TORS for resecting sellar tumors in 2016, with some modifications to the above approach [60]. They prospectively selected four patients to undergo TORS for resection of a sellar tumor with suprasellar and cystic components using three arms of the da Vinci Si robot (Intuitive Surgical; Sunnyvale, California, USA). All patients had an oral aperture of at least 38 mm. Successful TORS requires a normal oral aperture generally ranging from 38.9 mm to 45 mm [34]. With an endotracheal tube in the left labial commissure and robotic arms at the head of the patient, an 8.5-mm 30° endoscope was inserted into the mouth behind the posterior edge of the hard palate to identify the cavum landmarks, choanae, and posterior nasal septum superiorly and eustachian tubes laterally. EndoWrist instruments (5 mm) in the two arms were introduced into the mouth and used to dissect a U-shaped flap along the hard palate, which was then positioned along the right choana for the sphenoidal approach. The key point defined as the junction between the vomer and sphenoid was identified and the robotic arms were removed to allow for drilling, but the endoscopic arm was left in place. The sphenoid sinus was opened inferiorly and expanded with a combination of drilling, robotic arm instruments, and Kerrison rongeurs. The dura was opened with a flexible fiber CO_2 laser (Lumenis Be Ltd., Yokneam, Israel) along with robotic instruments. The tumor was resected, and a mucosal flap was replaced [60].

The literature describes few complications associated with TORS for anterior skull base surgery, probably because only a limited number of surgical procedures have been performed on patients. As with any intradural anterior skull base procedure, there is an inherent risk for cerebrospinal fluid (CSF) leakage [60]. Additionally, there is a hypothetical risk for velopharyngeal or velopalatine insufficiency owing to scar contracture, and a risk of oronasal fistula formation; however, neither of these has been reported in the literature for robotic anterior skull base surgery [51, 60]. More benign postoperative risks associated with TORS include dysphagia, temporomandibular joint pain, delayed otitis media, and sore throat [61, 62].

Despite the successful use of TORS to access the anterior skull base and sellar/parasellar regions, significant limitations to this single port approach limit its generalizability. Patients without normal oral apertures are not amenable to this procedure. The steep angles of the anterior skull base make the da Vinci robotic arms difficult to maneuver cephalad to gain further anterior access to the anterior skull base. Cadaveric and clinical studies have demonstrated that an endonasal endoscopic approach complementing TORS allows for improved visibility in areas such as the infratemporal fossa, nasopharynx, clivus, and craniovertebral junction [63]. Finally, this is not a strictly robotic procedure because an assistant is required at the bedside to assist with some tasks such as drilling.

5.3.1.2 Robotic Surgery

The endoscopic endonasal approach has become the workhorse for neurosurgical minimal access to the anterior skull base and sellar/parasellar regions. Despite this, the transition to a direct robotic endonasal approach has been difficult because the restrictions of nostril diameter and angle lead to a narrow funnel effect [52]. A pure transnasal approach with the Medrobotic Flex system (Medrobotics Corp.; Raynham, Massachusetts, USA) was described by Schuler and colleagues in 2015 [64]. This system is a surgeon-controlled flexible robotic endoscope with a high-definition camera and six LED light sources at the tip providing 3D working space and flexibility of up to 180° (Figs. 5.2, 5.3, and 5.4).

There are two working channels on either side of the endoscope allowing for delivery of instruments and triangulation of tools in the working space. The diameter at the tip is 15x17 mm and the maximum distance the endoscope can travel is 17 cm. Owing to the restrictions of nostril diameter, partial midface degloving, and partial nasal septectomy were needed to allow the Flex Systems endoscope to be placed in the nasal cavity [64].

Although adequate visualization of the sinus system and skull base is feasible, this procedure is invasive as it requires partial midfacial degloving and, potentially, piriform ostetomies. Binasal approaches could be feasible, but computer modeling demonstrates that the optimal angle between two robotic tools transnasally at the skull base is at least 20°; however, the current working angle with the da Vinci robot (Intuitive Surgical; Sunnyvale, California, USA) is only 14.7°. Therefore, this approach is best used with a combined transorbital or transmaxillary approach [34, 65]. Novel robotic endoscope holders have also been employed in transnasal approaches for pituitary pathologies, the goal being to reduce the physical strain on

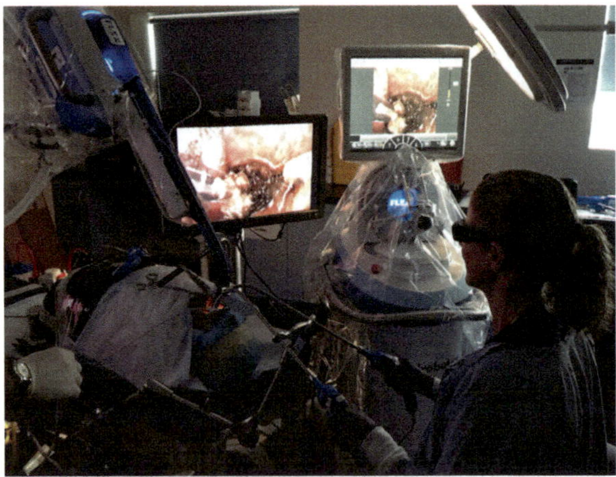

Fig. 5.2 Author Raewyn Campbell shows a transoral approach to the skull base using the Medrobotics Flex robot (Medrobotics Corp.; Raynham, Massachusetts, USA), demonstrating the position of the surgeon and favorable ergonomic posture

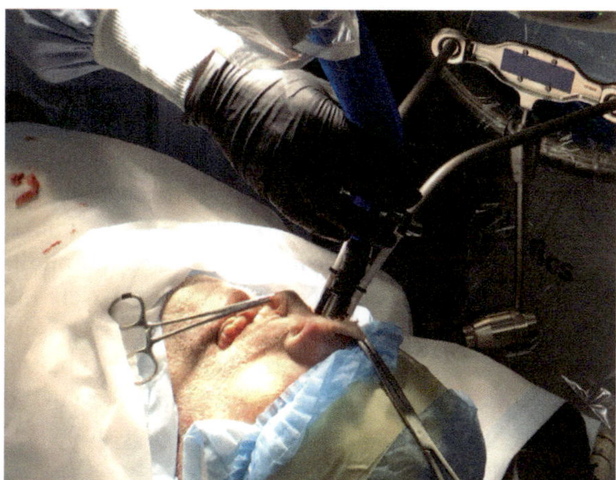

Fig. 5.3 Demonstration of the transnasal approach to the skull base using the Medrobotics Flex robot (Medrobotics Corp.; Raynham, Massachusetts, USA). A modified Weber Ferguson incision was required, and the bony piriform aperture was drilled to access the full nasal cavity and skull base

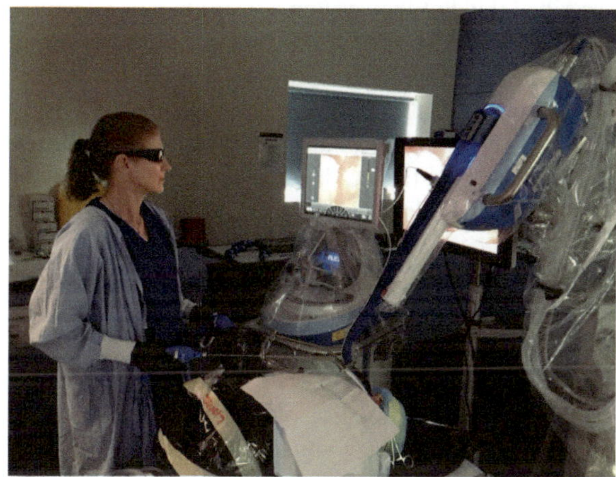

Fig. 5.4 Another option for positioning using the Medrobotic Flex robot (Medrobotics Corp.; Raynham, Massachusetts, USA) transnasally

surgeons while freeing up an additional hand for them [50, 66]. However, as mentioned above, the limitations of space remain.

5.3.1.3 Transorbital/Supraorbital Robotic Approaches

The robotic supraorbital keyhole approach to the anterior skull base using the da Vinci robot (Intuitive Surgical; Sunnyvale, California, USA) has only been described in cadavers [67]. The robot was positioned 30° relative to the body on the right side of the head, which was secured in 10–15° of extension. After a supraorbital craniotomy, a 0° and 30° upward-facing stereoscopic endoscope was placed through the keyhole to visualize the anatomy prior to the placement of the da Vinci robotic arms. Self-retaining retractors with brain ribbons were used. The surgeon remained at the non-sterile robotic console throughout the procedure. The dura was opened with robotic curved scissors and the right frontal lobe was retracted with a self-retaining snake retractor. Brain relaxation was achieved by CSF release. The optico-carotid cistern was opened with the robotic arm, allowing the optic nerve, optic chiasm, internal carotid artery, and oculomotor nerve to be visualized. An EndoWrist suction/irrigator along with Potts scissors was used to open the Sylvian fissure. The authors could navigate the deep narrow corridor, and after the M1 segment was incised, three sutures were placed relatively quickly and easily to close the defect.

The chiasmatic cistern was then approached and opened using the robot. The 0° endoscope was used to visualize the sellar region. EndoWrist instruments were advanced into the pre-chiasmatic space and the pituitary stalk, gland, tuberculum sellae, and contralateral internal carotid artery were identified. The lamina terminalis was opened, the anterior cerebral artery was dissected to the junction of the A1 and A2 segments, and the recurrent artery of Heubner was identified. The origins of the posterior communicating and anterior choroidal arteries were also visualized. Robotic tools could not perform clip ligation at this point, so a manual clip applier was used to place an aneurysm clip [67].

This mono-portal approach is not uncontroversial. Marcus and colleagues described the da Vinci system's instruments and cameras as overly large, unable to provide adequate visualization, and unsafe for a 25-mm keyhole craniotomy [68]. Therefore, the supraorbital approach could be best as a combined approach with multiple portals. The development of more fine-tuned tools with smaller footprints could make the transorbital approach more feasible, as demonstrated by Faulkner and colleagues in their cadaveric feasibility study using the Versius surgical system (CMR Surgical; Cambridge, UK) [69].

5.3.2 Multi-Portal/Combined Approaches

5.3.2.1 Cervical Transoral Robotic Surgery

To circumvent the limitation of oral aperture size, which leads to a narrow angle for robotic arm access and limits the number of robotic arms accessing the anterior skull base to two or three, cervical transoral robotic surgery (C-TORS) was developed [55]. This combined approach makes it possible to achieve robotic access to the skull base from the cribriform plate and fovea ethmoidalis to the sellar and parasellar regions, clivus, infratemporal and pterygopalatine fossae, and the nasopharynx. O'Malley first described C-TORS approaches in cadavers in 2007 [55]. Using the da Vinci robot (Intuitive Surgical; Sunnyvale, California, USA), a 3D camera was placed transorally. A 3-mm incision was made bilaterally along the posterior border of the submandibular gland. Plastic introducers and round-tip dilators were passed blindly in a circular motion until the camera visualized them intraorally. Injury was avoided by tenting the oral mucosa at the lateral hypopharyngeal region by the round tip dilators and then inspecting the transparent mucosa to determine whether critical structures were trapped by the introducer tip. The mucosa was incised by monopolar cautery. Metal trocars were then placed in the field to admit the passage of 5 mm instruments. To verify that no neurovascular and airway structures had been injured during introducer and trocar passage, the cadaver neck was opened and visually inspected. The TORS approach was performed as described above. Because the increased angles between the robotic arms meant they were no longer constricted by the oral aperture, the anterior and middle skull base including the sella, parasellar, and suprasellar regions could be visualized thanks to the increased maneuverability of instrumentation [55]. A modification by Dallan and colleagues involved endonasal instead of transoral visualization [70], which also provided access to the posterior skull base.

C-TORS provides adequate access to the anterior skull base but is significantly invasive because the trocars are passed blindly through the neck. While the trocars are being passed, injury to critical structures such as the airway and neurovascular bundles in addition to soft tissue destruction could lead to airway collapse, hematoma formation, compressive edema, and injury to the lower cranial nerves. Also, as with TORS, there is a risk for velopalatine insufficiency. In view of these risks, the C-TORS approach has not advanced beyond the preclinical phase of testing.

5.3.2.2 Suprahyoid-Transoral Robotic Approaches

The suprahyoid-transoral approach was described in cadavers by McCool and colleagues as an alternative to the C-TORS approach [56]. A 2–0 silk suture was used to pull the tongue anteriorly and the palate was retracted with a 10-french red rubber catheter placed transnasally and pulled through the mouth. The cadavers underwent nasal intubation to simulate live operative technique. A 1-cm cannula was inserted via a blunt introducer through a 15-mm midline incision at the level of the hyoid bone. With a finger at the base of the tongue, the cannula was guided blindly to the oropharynx via the vallecula. A bite block was placed in the mouth ipsilateral to the side of dissection. The 30° camera of the da Vinci robot (Intuitive Surgical; Sunnyvale, California, USA) and a second robotic arm were placed transorally on the contralateral side. Soft tissue dissection with incision of the posterior tonsillar pillar proceeded superiorly along the salpingopharyngeal fold 5 mm inferior to the torus tubarius. The superior pharyngeal muscle and lateral aponeurotic sheath of the medial pterygoid were divided. The lingual and inferior alveolar branches of cranial nerve V_3 were identified and dissected superiorly to the foramen ovale and the middle meningeal artery was also identified. Dissection proceeded posteriorly to the jugular foramen, internal jugular vein, and lower cranial nerves (IX–XII). One robotic arm and one camera were placed transorally, minimizing the mobility limitations from the robotic arm angles in approaching the anterior skull base [59].

The risks associated with the suprahyoid-transoral approach include hypoglossal nerve injury. This could be mitigated by placing the trocar in the midline as the hypoglossal nerves are lateral. Pre-epiglottic swelling and supraglottis are other risks that could require long-term intubation or tracheostomy [56, 59].

5.3.2.3 Endonasal Transmaxillary Approach

The combined endonasal transmaxillary approach as an approach to the anterior skull base in four cadavers was first described by Hanna and colleagues in 2007 [54]. They performed bilateral sublabial incisions, and soft tissue flaps were elevated to the level of the infraorbital nerves superiorly and nasal piriform aperture medially. Wide anterior maxillary Caldwell-Luc antrostomies were performed.

Wide middle meatal antrostomies and a posterior nasal septectomy were also performed to allow the three arms of the da Vinci robot (Intuitive Surgical; Sunnyvale, California, USA) to be introduced. The camera arm port with a 5-mm dual channel endoscope and a dual charge-coupled device camera for 3D visualization was placed in the nostril and the right and left surgical arm ports were placed in the respective anterior and middle antrostomies to the nasal cavities. Endoscopic anterior and posterior ethmoidectomies could be performed with or without resection of the superior and middle turbinates. The robotic arms were manipulated to perform a sphenoidectomy and expose the planum sphenoidale and sella turcica. Further anterior skull base dissection was performed to resect the cribriform plate, create a dural opening, and repair the opening with sutures [54].

In 2013, Blanco and colleagues expanded on the combined endonasal transmaxillary approach with the da Vinci robot (Intuitive Surgical; Sunnyvale, California, USA) in response to the constraints of limited nostril diameter [71]. A rhinoplasty-type transcolumellar incision was performed and Lega's technique was used to make marginal incisions along the anterior and posterior margins of the medial crural cartilage to release the medial crural footplates. This allowed the skin below the transcolumellar incision to be freed from the medial crural cartilages, and also expanded the nostrils while reflecting the nasal tip superiorly to create an increased range in the cranial-caudal plane for the endoscope. The inferior turbinates were outfractured and the nostril was expanded in the horizontal plane by a partial septectomy [71].

Despite expanding the nasal corridor, a separate transmaxillary osteoplastic window was needed for instrument mobilization. With a sublabial incision from the central incisor to the third molar, and partial facial degloving with elevation of the soft tissue of the cheek to the level of the inferior orbital rim, an osteoplastic window was removed while the infraorbital nerve was preserved. Robotic arms were positioned at 30° and the posterior and medial maxillary walls were resected to achieve exposure to the nasal cavity. The osteoplastic transmaxillary window enabled up to four 5-mm instruments to be placed in the operative field without obscuring visualization or impairing the mobility of the robotic arms. In the infratemporal fossa, the maxillary and middle meningeal arteries, cranial nerves V_2 and V_3, lateral pterygoid, foramen rotundum, and foramen ovale were identified. Anterior skull base dissection could be performed with access to the posterior ethmoid, sphenoid, sella turcica, and suprasellar and parasellar regions. Stereotactic navigation to verify surgical position involved a Medtronic AxIEM emitter (Medtronic; Minneapolis, Minnesota, USA) and the da Vinci Tilpro interfaced with it. A pedicle septal flap was sutured by the robot to close the anterior skull base defect [71].

Despite the greater access to the anterior skull base, this combined approach is invasive. The endonasal transmaxillary approach requires a significant expansion of the nasal corridor and does not provide access to the anterior ethmoid bone or middle meatus [71].

5.3.2.4 Transcranial Robotic Approach

The ROSA—Robotic Stereotactic System (Zimmer Biomet; Warsaw, Indiana, USA)—is a computer-controlled robotic arm used for stereotactic frameless surgery. It has built-in system software used to implant brain electrodes and for laser interstitial thermal therapy (LITT), catheter placement, frameless stereotactic biopsy, and endoscopic third ventriculostomies [72–75]. After the trajectory to the lesion is planned, the patient is positioned in a Mayfield head holder fixed to the ROSA. The fixed orientation of the head allows for precise robotic stereotaxy. The registration is semiautomated and built into the ROSA system. It uses a laser at the end of the robotic arm to scan the patients' facial contours and relate them to prior 3D high-definition CT or MRI volumetric images. The arm can either be automatically driven or manually adjusted along the axis of the trajectory to achieve a comfortable working distance. Miller and colleagues described the placement of depth electrodes using the ROSA system in eleven pediatric patients with no major complications, and performing biopsy and/or LITT on six patients [72]. Two patients had lesions in the anterior cranial fossa that the ROSA robot accessed for biopsy, stereo-EEG, and LITT. A similar robotic stereotactic system is the RONNA G3 system, which has been used clinically for precise localization during brain biopsy [76].

5.4 Limitations of Robotic Surgery in the Anterior Cranial Fossa

Robotic anterior skull base surgery is limited not only by the complex anatomy and steep angles of the anterior skull base but also by the robotic devices and instrumentation available. The narrow funnel effect, being the minimum angle required between robotic tools to allow for function, is a limitation that currently available robots find difficult to overcome. Bly and colleagues used computer modeling and Artificial Intelligence (AI) tools to analyze the approach trajectories, angles between robotic tools, and distances to skull base lesions in cadavers [65]. These were then tested using the da Vinci robot (Intuitive Surgical; Sunnyvale, California, USA) and Raven robotic systems (BioRobotics Laboratory; Seattle, Washington, USA). They identified increased collisions between robotic arms when the portals were close to each other. Additionally, steep approach vectors to the anterior skull base limited the use of robotic surgical portals. The addition of more portals improved the funnel effect and also improved robotic arm maneuverability.

Robotic arm and instrument size limit maneuverability through working portals [34]. This makes robotic surgery technically feasible in cadaveric studies but potentially unsafe in the clinical setting. Current robots cannot drill autonomously and provide limited haptic feedback. Finally, there is a significant lack of instruments with an intraoperative navigation component for anterior skull base surgery in currently developed robots [77]. This will need to be addressed in future iterations of robots to provide the surgeon with accurate navigation to skull base lesions.

5.5 Future Directions

Robotic surgery, particularly for anterior skull base surgery, has made major strides since its original adoption. However, many advances are still needed for robotic approaches to become as commonplace as endoscope-based techniques. Many of the improvements outlined below relate to robotic surgery generally while others are more specific to neurosurgery.

1. *Miniaturization of Instruments and Increased Instrument Flexibility:* One major pitfall in adopting robotic platforms for use in the anterior skull base has been the size and rigidity of available instruments [34, 65]. This becomes obvious when we consider that many currently employed instruments were not originally intended for use in the small cavities/passageways common in neurosurgery, especially skull base surgery. Thus, one of the biggest advances in the adoption of robotic platforms for anterior skull base surgery would be to create tailored instruments that are small and flexible to operate within a confined environment. A perfect example is the development of concentric tube robots that specifically address the narrow confines of skull base surgery [78]. Extended use of surgical trocars [79] and synergistic collaboration between surgeons and engineers aimed at merging micro-technologies with surgical robotics [80] and improving robot design will eventually lay the foundations for a stepwise advance in the use of robots in skull base surgery [81].
2. *Drilling Capabilities:* In conjunction with the points discussed above regarding the development of new instruments, current robotic platforms also lack drilling capabilities because they do not have the necessary tools or the distal robotic arm strength to stabilize drilling through thick bone. Current TORS performed for anterior cranial fossa access relies on handheld drills [60]. Studies are underway to develop drilling instruments that have simultaneous force feedback [82, 83].
3. *Suturing Capabilities:* Although the adoption of robotic surgery in the confines of skull base surgery allows for more instrument articulation during suturing than endoscopic/microscopic-based techniques, suturing capabilities can still be improved. The most obvious improvement would be force-feedback capabilities, allowing for more fine-tuned handling of the delicate sutures often employed, for example, in vascular procedures [84]. However, the potential for semi- or even full automation of suturing using specialized instruments is more interesting. Many publications have assessed the ability to automate this process in both laparoscopic and robotic surgeries [85–87]. Novel needle-grasping tools have also been developed for adaptation to current robotic surgical platforms [86, 87].
4. *Haptic Feedback:* One of the major drawbacks of any present-day robotic surgical system is the lack of haptic feedback to guide surgeons in the intraoperative manipulation of tissue or other materials [88]. The delicate nature of nerves and blood vessels in anterior skull base surgery means that haptic feedback will be pivotal if safe operations such as tumor resection (regardless of stiffness) or aneurysm clipping are to be performed [89–91]. The utility and feasibility of

incorporating such feedback have been investigated, and it is under development for use in next-generation robotic platforms [92].

5. *Integration of Intraoperative Navigation:* Neurosurgery and skull base surgery, more than any other surgical sub-specialty, depend on a deep understanding of anatomy and on intraoperative imaging navigation to ensure accurate localization [93]. Real-time imaging navigation has many applications, ranging from stereotactic neurosurgery to tumor margin determination and aneurysm clipping [93, 94]. Incorporating real-time instrument navigation with robotic platforms would truly be groundbreaking, and its feasibility has been demonstrated for skull base surgery in cadavers [95]. Newer technology relying on electromagnetic fields for instrument detection promises great adaptability with techniques such as TORS, since no direct line of sight is needed for navigation, and instrument footprint is minimal [96].
6. *Employing Artificial Intelligence:* Recent developments in machine learning have allowed computer vision to be applied to surgery, the computer being able to interpret operative images or video reliably [97, 98]. Computer vision promises the real-time ability to predict important regional anatomy and the next steps in an operation, and even to distinguish healthy from tumor tissue when brain and skull base tumors are to be resected [99–103]. Incorporating such a tool into robotic platforms, and even augmented reality, could provide for a seamless operating experience tailored to each operation and surgeon.
7. *Improving Affordability:* Needless to say, robotic operating platforms have yet to become affordable. System costs are often in the millions of dollars, not including annual maintenance fees or instrument costs [104]. Therefore, access to surgical robotic systems remains limited for many institutions. As more platforms are developed and robotics spread more widely around the world, costs will eventually decrease.
8. *Improving Platform Ergonomics:* Current robotic operating platforms occupy significant space within operating rooms. Also, they often require personnel familiar with the systems to help with setup and management [104, 105]. There is therefore room for improvement in the design of special operating rooms to accommodate robotic systems, and even the design of the systems themselves, ultimately allowing for small footprints and greater ease of use for hospital staff interacting with the modules.
9. *Tele-Surgery Applications:* As robotic surgical platforms are adopted, the ability for providers to perform tele-surgery has become a reality. The first remote operation was a laparoscopic cholecystectomy performed in 2001, with an uncomplicated recovery by the patient [106]. Unfortunately, applications in neurosurgery have remained extremely limited [107]. Tele-robotic spinal surgery of the thoracic/lumbar spine has been demonstrated in the literature [108]. A feasibility study examining tele-surgical removal of a phantom pituitary tumor in a cadaver demonstrated minimal video latency over the 800-km distance and no observable differences for the surgeon performing the task locally and then remotely [109]. Tele-intervention has also been adopted in percutaneous coronary intervention and could perhaps be extrapolated to treating strokes, as demonstrated in

preclinical models by Britz et al. [110–112]. Improvements in network technology, e.g., widespread adoption of 5G, and network security, e.g., blockchain-based frameworks, could allow for more seamless integration of tele-surgical practices [113].

5.6 Conclusions

Robotic platforms for operating on anterior cranial fossa pathologies remain in their infancy. Although several robotic platforms and anatomical approaches have been shown to be feasible at various levels, there has been minimal extrapolation to clinical settings. However, as with any new surgical technique, the development of more refined tools promises greater applicability. More importantly, the eventual adoption of robotic approaches to the anterior cranial fossa promises greater operative ease and potentially better patient outcomes, akin to the leaps accompanying the first adoption of microsurgical or endoscopic approaches in neurosurgery and skull base surgery.

References

1. Mazzoni A, Krengli M. Historical development of the treatment of skull base tumours. Rep Pract Oncol Radiother. 2016;21(4):319–24.
2. Yang C, et al. Transsphenoidal versus transcranial approach for treatment of tuberculum Sellae Meningiomas: a systematic review and meta-analysis of comparative studies. Sci Rep. 2019;9(1):4882.
3. Abu-Ghanem S, Fliss DM. Surgical approaches to resection of anterior skull base and paranasal sinuses tumors. Balkan Med J. 2013;30(2):136–41.
4. Chi JH, et al. Extended bifrontal craniotomy for midline anterior fossa meningiomas: minimization of retraction-related edema and surgical outcomes. Neurosurgery. 2006;59(4 Suppl 2):ONS426–33. discussion ONS433-4
5. Liu P, et al. Effect of clipping anterior communicating artery aneurysms via pterional approach contralateral to supply of dominant blood: report of 15 patients. Int J Clin Exp Med. 2015;8(2):1912–7.
6. Aso K, et al. Microsurgical clipping for anterior communicating artery aneurysm associated with the accessory anterior cerebral artery via the pterional approach. Surg Neurol Int. 2018;9:120.
7. Musleh W, Sonabend AM, Lesniak MS. Role of craniotomy in the management of pituitary adenomas and sellar/parasellar tumors. Expert Rev Anticancer Ther. 2006;6(Suppl 9):S79–83.
8. Kiyofuji S, et al. Anterior interhemispheric approach for clipping of subcallosal distal anterior cerebral artery aneurysms: case series and technical notes. Neurosurg Rev. 2020;43(2):801–6.
9. Sherif C, et al. A management algorithm for cerebrospinal fluid leak associated with anterior skull base fractures: detailed clinical and radiological follow-up. Neurosurg Rev. 2012;35(2):227–37. discussion 237–8
10. Di Ieva A, et al. The comprehensive AOCMF classification: Skull Base and cranial vault fractures - level 2 and 3 tutorial. Craniomaxillofac Trauma Reconstr. 2014;7(Suppl 1):S103–13.
11. Morales-Valero SF, et al. Craniotomy for anterior cranial fossa meningiomas: historical overview. Neurosurg Focus. 2014;36(4):E14.

12. Schmidt RF, Choudry OJ, Takkellapati R, Ely JA, Couldwell WT, Liu JK. Hermann Schloffer and the origin of transphenoidal pituitary surgery. Neurosurg Focus. 2012;33(2):E5.
13. Uluc K, Kujoth GC, Baskaya MK. Operating microscopes: past, present, and future. Neurosurg Focus. 2009;27(3):E4.
14. Gelberman RH. Microsurgery and the development of the operating microscope. Contemp Surg. 1978;13(6):43–6.
15. Yaşargil MG, Abernathey CD. Microneurosurgery of CNS tumors. Thieme; 1996.
16. Comtois R, et al. The clinical and endocrine outcome to transsphenoidal microsurgery of nonsecreting pituitary adenomas. Cancer. 1991;68(4):860–6.
17. Di Ieva A, et al. A journey into the technical evolution of neuroendoscopy. World Neurosurg. 2014;82(6):e777–89.
18. Apuzzo MLJ, Heifetz MD, Weiss MH, Kurze T. Neurosurgical endoscopy using the side-viewing telescope. J Neurosurg. 1977;46:398–400.J.
19. Jho HD, Carrau RL. Endoscopy assisted transsphenoidal surgery for pituitary adenoma. Technical note. Acta Neurochir (Wien). 1996;138(12):1416–25.
20. Cusimano MD, Fenton RS. The technique for endoscopic pituitary tumor removal. Neurosurg Focus. 1996;1(1):e1. discussion 1p following e3.
21. Chibbaro S, et al. Endoscopic Transorbital approaches to anterior and middle cranial fossa: exploring the potentialities of a modified lateral Retrocanthal approach. World Neurosurg. 2021;150:e74–80.
22. Khan DZ, et al. The endoscope-assisted supraorbital "keyhole" approach for anterior skull base meningiomas: an updated meta-analysis. Acta Neurochir. 2021;163(3):661–76.
23. Zada G. Editorial: the endoscopic keyhole supraorbital approach. Neurosurg Focus. 2014;37(4):E21.
24. Perneczky A, Fries G. Endoscope-assisted brain surgery: part 1--evolution, basic concept, and current technique. Neurosurgery. 1998;42(2):219–24. discussion 224–5.
25. Fries G, Perneczky A. Endoscope-assisted brain surgery: part 2--analysis of 380 procedures. Neurosurgery. 1998;42(2):226–31. discussion 231–2
26. Wilson DA, et al. The supraorbital endoscopic approach for tumors. World Neurosurg. 2014;82(1–2):e243–56.
27. Shao D, et al. Keyhole approach for clipping anterior circulation aneurysms: clinical outcomes and technical note. Front Surg. 2021;8:783557.
28. Castlen JP, et al. The extended, transnasal, transsphenoidal approach for anterior skull base meningioma: considerations in patient selection. Pituitary. 2017;20(5):561–8.
29. Guo S, et al. A meta-analysis of endoscopic vs. microscopic Transsphenoidal surgery for non-functioning and functioning pituitary adenomas: comparisons of efficacy and safety. Front Neurol. 2021;12:614382.
30. Moller MW, et al. Endoscopic vs. microscopic transsphenoidal pituitary surgery: a single Centre study. Sci Rep. 2020;10(1):21942.
31. Fathalla H, et al. Cerebrospinal fluid leaks in extended endoscopic transsphenoidal surgery: covering all the angles. Neurosurg Rev. 2017;40(2):309–18.
32. Fathalla H, et al. Endoscopic versus microscopic approach for surgical treatment of acromegaly. Neurosurg Rev. 2015;38(3):541–8. discussion 548–9
33. O'Malley BW Jr, et al. Comparison of endoscopic and microscopic removal of pituitary adenomas: single-surgeon experience and the learning curve. Neurosurg Focus. 2008;25(6):E10.
34. Campbell RG, Harvey RJ. How close are we to anterior robotic skull base surgery? Curr Opin Otolaryngol Head Neck Surg. 2021;29(1):44–52.
35. de Almeida JR, Carvalho F, Vaz Guimaraes Filho F, et al. Comparison of endoscopic endonasal and bifrontal craniotomy approaches for olfactory groove meningiomas: a matched pair analysis of outcomes and frontal lobe changes on MRI. J Clin Neurosci. 2015;22(11):1733–41.
36. Rimmer J, et al. Endoscopic sinus surgery and musculoskeletal symptoms. Rhinology. 2016;54(2):105–10.

37. Little RM, et al. Occupational hazards of endoscopic surgery. Int Forum Allergy Rhinol. 2012;2(3):212–6.
38. Di Ieva A. Training in skull base surgery: a holistic perspective. J Neurosurg Sci. 2017;61(6):690–1.
39. Tschabitscher M, Di Ieva A. Practical guidelines for setting up an endoscopic/skull base cadaver laboratory. World Neurosurg. 2013;79(2 Suppl):S16 e1–7.
40. Di Ieva A, Tschabitscher M. Letter to the editor regarding the exoscope in neurosurgery: an innovative point of view. A systematic review of the technical, surgical, and educational aspects. World Neurosurg. 2019;127:652.
41. Mamelak AN, Nobuto T, Berci G. Initial clinical experience with a high-definition exoscope system for microneurosurgery. Neurosurgery. 2010;67(2):476–83.
42. Krishnan KG, Scholler K, Uhl E. Application of a compact high-definition exoscope for illumination and magnification in high-precision surgical procedures. World Neurosurg. 2017;97:652–60.
43. Gassie K, Wijesekera O, Chaichana KL. Minimally invasive tubular retractor-assisted biopsy and resection of subcortical intra-axial gliomas and other neoplasms. J Neurosurg Sci. 2018;62(6):682–9.
44. Khalessi AA, et al. First-in-man clinical experience using a high-definition 3-dimensional exoscope system for microneurosurgery. Oper Neurosurg (Hagerstown). 2019;16(6):717–25.
45. Iwata T, et al. Microsurgery "under the eaves" using ORBEYE: a case of Dural arteriovenous fistula of the anterior cranial fossa. World Neurosurg. 2020;138:178–81.
46. Rosler J, et al. Clinical implementation of a 3D4K-exoscope (Orbeye) in microneurosurgery. Neurosurg Rev. 2022;45(1):627–35.
47. Klinger DR, et al. Microsurgical clipping of an anterior communicating artery aneurysm using a novel robotic visualization tool in lieu of the binocular operating microscope: operative video. Oper Neurosurg (Hagerstown). 2018;14(1):26–8.
48. Montemurro N, et al. The exoscope in neurosurgery: an overview of the current literature of intraoperative use in brain and spine surgery. J Clin Med. 2021;11(1)
49. Campbell RG. Robotic surgery of the anterior skull base. Int Forum Allergy Rhinol. 2019;9(12):1508–14.
50. Pangal DJ, et al. Robotic and robot-assisted skull base neurosurgery: systematic review of current applications and future directions. Neurosurg Focus. 2022;52(1):E15.
51. Elsabeh R, et al. Cranial neurosurgical robotics. Br J Neurosurg. 2021;35(5):532–40.
52. Heuermann M, Michael AP, Crosby DL. Robotic Skull Base surgery. Otolaryngol Clin N Am. 2020;53(6):1077–89.
53. Trevillot V, et al. Robotic endoscopic sinus and skull base surgery: review of the literature and future prospects. Eur Ann Otorhinolaryngol Head Neck Dis. 2013;130(4):201–7.
54. Hanna EY, et al. Robotic endoscopic surgery of the skull base: a novel surgical approach. Arch Otolaryngol Head Neck Surg. 2007;133(12):1209–14.
55. O'Malley BW Jr, Weinstein GS. Robotic anterior and midline skull base surgery: preclinical investigations. Int J Radiat Oncol Biol Phys. 2007;69(2 Suppl):S125–8.
56. McCool RR, et al. Robotic surgery of the infratemporal fossa utilizing novel suprahyoid port. Laryngoscope. 2010;120(9):1738–43.
57. Schneider JS, et al. Robotic surgery for the sinuses and skull base: what are the possibilities and what are the obstacles? Curr Opin Otolaryngol Head Neck Surg. 2013;21(1):11–6.
58. Hintschich CA, et al. A third hand to the surgeon: the use of an endoscope holding arm in endonasal sinus surgery and well beyond. Eur Arch Otorhinolaryngol. 2022;279(4):1891–8.
59. Lee JY, et al. Transoral robotic surgery of the skull base: a cadaver and feasibility study. ORL J Otorhinolaryngol Relat Spec. 2010;72(4):181–7.
60. Chauvet D, et al. Transoral robotic surgery for sellar tumors: first clinical study. J Neurosurg. 2017;127(4):941–8.
61. Hay A, et al. Complications following transoral robotic surgery (TORS): a detailed institutional review of complications. Oral Oncol. 2017;67:160–6.
62. Cammaroto G, et al. Alternative applications of TransOral robotic surgery (TORS): a systematic review. J Clin Med. 2020;9(1)

63. Carrau RL, et al. Combined transoral robotic surgery and endoscopic endonasal approach for the resection of extensive malignancies of the skull base. Head Neck. 2013;35(11):E351–8.
64. Schuler PJ, et al. A single-port operator-controlled flexible endoscope system for endoscopic skull base surgery. HNO. 2015;63(3):189–94.
65. Bly RA, et al. Multiportal robotic access to the anterior cranial fossa: a surgical and engineering feasibility study. Otolaryngol Head Neck Surg. 2013;149(6):940–6.
66. Zappa F, et al. Hybrid robotics for endoscopic Transnasal Skull Base surgery: single-Centre case series. Oper Neurosurg (Hagerstown). 2021;21(6):426–35.
67. Hong WC, et al. Robotic skull base surgery via supraorbital keyhole approach: a cadaveric study. Neurosurgery. 2013;72(Suppl 1):33–8.
68. Marcus HJ, et al. da Vinci robot-assisted keyhole neurosurgery: a cadaver study on feasibility and safety. Neurosurg Rev. 2015;38(2):367–71. discussion 371
69. Faulkner J, et al. Combined robotic transorbital and transnasal approach to the nasopharynx and anterior skull base: feasibility study. Clin Otolaryngol. 2020;45(4):630–3.
70. Dallan I, et al. Combined transnasal transcervical robotic dissection of posterior skull base: feasibility in a cadaveric model. Rhinology. 2012;50(2):165–70.
71. Blanco RG, Boahene K. Robotic-assisted skull base surgery: preclinical study. J Laparoendosc Adv Surg Tech A. 2013;23(9):776–82.
72. Miller BA, et al. Applications of a robotic stereotactic arm for pediatric epilepsy and neurooncology surgery. J Neurosurg Pediatr. 2017;20(4):364–70.
73. Hoshide R, et al. Robot-assisted endoscopic third ventriculostomy: institutional experience in 9 patients. J Neurosurg Pediatr. 2017;20(2):125–33.
74. Alan N, et al. Robotic stereotactic assistance (ROSA) utilization for minimally invasive placement of Intraparenchymal hematoma and intraventricular catheters. World Neurosurg. 2017;108:996 e7–996 e10.
75. Nelson JH, et al. Robotic stereotactic assistance (ROSA) for pediatric epilepsy: a single-center experience of 23 consecutive cases. Children (Basel). 2020;7(8)
76. Dlaka D, et al. Brain biopsy performed with the RONNA G3 system: a case study on using a novel robotic navigation device for stereotactic neurosurgery. Int J Med Robot. 2018;14(1)
77. Caversaccio M, Zheng G, Nolte LP. Computer-aided surgery of the paranasal sinuses and the anterior skull base. HNO. 2008;56(4):376–8. 780–2
78. Bergeles C, et al. Concentric tube robot design and optimization based on task and anatomical constraints. IEEE Trans Robot. 2015;31(1):67–84.
79. Cusimano MD, et al. Canula-assisted endoscopy in bi-portal transphenoidal cranial base surgery: technical note. Acta Neurochir. 2013;155(5):909–11.
80. Di Ieva A. Microtechnologies in neurosurgery. Proc Inst Mech Eng H. 2010;224(6):797–800.
81. Chalongwongse S, Chumnanvej S, Suthakorn J. Analysis of Endonasal endoscopic Transsphenoidal (EET) surgery pathway and workspace for path guiding robot design. Asian J Surg. 2019;42(8):814–22.
82. Sang H, et al. A new surgical drill instrument with force sensing and force feedback for robotically assisted Otologic surgery. J Med Dev. 2017;11(3)
83. Torun Y, Ozturk A. A new breakthrough detection method for bone Drilling in Robotic Orthopedic Surgery with closed-loop control approach. Ann Biomed Eng. 2020;48(4):1218–29.
84. Bauernschmitt R, et al. Towards robotic heart surgery: introduction of autonomous procedures into an experimental surgical telemanipulator system. Int J Med Robot. 2005;1(3):74–9.
85. Saeidi H, et al. Autonomous robotic laparoscopic surgery for intestinal anastomosis. Sci Robot. 2022;7(62):eabj2908.
86. Leonard S, et al. Smart tissue anastomosis robot (STAR): a vision-guided robotics system for laparoscopic suturing. IEEE Trans Biomed Eng. 2014;61(4):1305–17.
87. Pedram SA, et al. Autonomous suturing framework and quantification using a cable-driven surgical robot. IEEE Trans Robot. 2021;37(2):404–17.
88. Francone A, et al. The effect of haptic feedback on efficiency and safety during Preretinal membrane peeling simulation. Transl Vis Sci Technol. 2019;8(4):2.

89. Di Ieva A, et al. Magnetic resonance elastography: a general overview of its current and future applications in brain imaging. Neurosurg Rev. 2010;33(2):137–45. discussion 145
90. Alaraj A, et al. Virtual reality cerebral aneurysm clipping simulation with real-time haptic feedback. Neurosurgery. 2015;11(Suppl 2):52–8.
91. Gmeiner M, et al. Virtual cerebral aneurysm clipping with real-time haptic force feedback in neurosurgical education. World Neurosurg. 2018;112:e313–23.
92. Aggravi M, et al. Hand-tool-tissue interaction forces in neurosurgery for haptic rendering. Med Biol Eng Comput. 2016;54(8):1229–41.
93. Orringer DA, Golby A, Jolesz F. Neuronavigation in the surgical management of brain tumors: current and future trends. Expert Rev Med Devices. 2012;9(5):491–500.
94. Schmid-Elsaesser R, et al. Neuronavigation based on CT angiography for surgery of intracranial aneurysms: primary experience with unruptured aneurysms. Minim Invasive Neurosurg. 2003;46(5):269–77.
95. Xia T, et al. An integrated system for planning, navigation and robotic assistance for skull base surgery. Int J Med Robot. 2008;4(4):321–30.
96. Tsang RK, Chung JCK. Adapting electromagnetic navigation system for Transoral robotic-assisted Skull Base surgery. Laryngoscope. 2020;130(8):1922–5.
97. Ward TM, et al. Computer vision in surgery. Surgery. 2021;169(5):1253–6.
98. Staartjes VE, et al. Machine vision for real-time intraoperative anatomic guidance: a proof-of-concept study in endoscopic pituitary surgery. Oper Neurosurg (Hagerstown). 2021;21(4):242–7.
99. Williams S, et al. Artificial intelligence in brain tumour surgery-an emerging paradigm. Cancers (Basel). 2021;13(19)
100. Fabelo H, et al. Deep learning-based framework for in vivo identification of glioblastoma tumor using hyperspectral images of human brain. Sensors (Basel). 2019;19(4)
101. Jiang C, et al. Rapid automated analysis of Skull Base tumor specimens using intraoperative optical imaging and artificial intelligence. Neurosurgery. 2022;90:758.
102. Hollon TC, et al. Rapid, label-free detection of diffuse glioma recurrence using intraoperative stimulated Raman histology and deep neural networks. Neuro-Oncology. 2021;23(1):144–55.
103. Hollon TC, et al. Near real-time intraoperative brain tumor diagnosis using stimulated Raman histology and deep neural networks. Nat Med. 2020;26(1):52–8.
104. Oliveira CM, et al. Robotic surgery in otolaryngology and head and neck surgery: a review. Minim Invasive Surg. 2012;2012:286563.
105. Kanji F, et al. Room size influences flow in robotic-assisted surgery. Int J Environ Res Public Health. 2021;18(15)
106. Marescaux J, et al. Transatlantic robot-assisted telesurgery. Nature. 2001;413(6854):379–80.
107. Xia SB, Lu QS. Development status of telesurgery robotic system. Chin J Traumatol. 2021;24(3):144–7.
108. Tian W, et al. Telerobotic spinal surgery based on 5G network: the first 12 cases. Neurospine. 2020;17(1):114–20.
109. Wirz R, et al. An experimental feasibility study on robotic endonasal telesurgery. Neurosurgery. 2015;76(4):479–84. discussion 484
110. Panesar SS, et al. Telerobotic stroke intervention: a novel solution to the care dissemination dilemma. J Neurosurg. 2019;132(3):971–8.
111. Patel TM, Shah SC, Pancholy SB. Long distance tele-robotic-assisted percutaneous coronary intervention: a report of first-in-human experience. EClinicalMedicine. 2019;14:53–8.
112. Britz GW, Tomas J, Lumsden A. Feasibility of robotic-assisted neurovascular interventions: initial experience in flow model and porcine model. Neurosurgery. 2020;86(2):309–14.
113. Gupta R, et al. Tactile-internet-based Telesurgery system for healthcare 4.0: an architecture, research challenges, and future directions. IEEE Netw. 2019;33(6):22–9.

6 Robotics for Approaches to the Mastoid/Mastoidectomy

Ahmet M. Tekin, Jaouad Abari, and Vedat Topsakal

6.1 The Evolution of Cochlear Implantation Surgery

Before discussing the developments of cochlear implantation surgery, it is necessary to describe the evolution of cochlear implant devices themselves. During the 1800s, Alessandro Volta showed that electrical stimulation of metal rods placed in a person's ear can produce an auditory sensation. The first single-channel cochlear implant device was introduced in 1972, and 12 years later the first multichannel cochlear implant device was devised, stimulating different parts of the cochlea at different frequencies [1]. With each stage in the development of cochlear implant devices, steps have been taken to improve sound and speech processing, thus achieving better speech recognition in patients [2].

One of the first cochlear implantation surgical techniques to be described is the posterior tympanoplasty or facial recess approach. This is considered one of the safest techniques, with a low risk of injuring the facial nerve. The first major steps in the operation are opening a retro-auricular skin flap and drilling the mastoid until the surgeon has approached the round window safely. After the round window is opened, the electrode array is inserted into the scala tympani of the cochlea [3]. Other techniques have been described in the past, differing in facial nerve injury risk, the risk of perforating the tympanic membrane, and electrode array insertion angles [4].

A. M. Tekin (✉)
HNO-Zentrum Polimed Caglan GmbH, Oberhausen, Germany

Department of Otorhinolaryngology Head and Neck Surgery, University Hospital UZ Brussel, Vrije Universiteit Brussel, Brussels, Belgium

J. Abari · V. Topsakal
Department of Otorhinolaryngology Head and Neck Surgery, University Hospital UZ Brussel, Vrije Universiteit Brussel, Brussels, Belgium
e-mail: abdeljaouad.abari@vub.be; Vedat.Topsakal@uzbrussel.be

M. M. Al-Salihi et al. (eds.), *Robotics in Skull-Base Surgery*,
https://doi.org/10.1007/978-3-031-38376-2_6

Following the advent of robotic surgery in general, robotically assisted cochlear implantation surgery (RACIS) has been developed in recent years. Implementing robotics into cochlear implantation surgery has made a minimally invasive round window approach without mastoidectomy a real possibility. More than 10 years have passed since RACIS was first described. RACIS could not have been developed without the progress afforded by image-guided technology. Pre- and intra-operative imaging makes it possible for the surgeon to plan a safe and efficient trajectory. A direct approach to the round window with a drill is only possible if the drill can pass safely through the space of the facial recess. This is the space between the facial nerve and the chorda tympani. It measures approximately 2.5–3.5 mm. Pre-clinical studies have shown that the facial recess space has to measure a minimum of 2.5 mm, and the spaces between the drill and the facial nerve/chorda tympani have to measure 0.4 mm and 0.3 mm, respectively, to avoid injury. It is understandable that the trajectory has to be planned carefully and accurately for a 1.8-mm drill to avoid these structures [5]. Because of small imaging inaccuracies, it is still necessary to ensure that the real trajectory does not deviate from the planned trajectory. Intra-operatively, the trajectory is double-checked using imaging and facial nerve monitoring to verify a safe distance from the facial nerve [4].

The first clinical application of RACIS is the drill passing through the space of the facial recess, approaching the round window. After having passed the facial recess robotically, the surgeon still had to open the round window manually and insert the electrode array under the microscope [6]. Recently, the HEARO- procedure has provided a step toward full automation of the surgery. With this procedure, the round window is opened autonomously because the drill opens its bony overhang (canonostomy), providing autonomous inner ear access [4].

6.2 The HEARO-Procedure

The HEARO-procedure has three main phases. The first phase is scanning and planning. After the patient's head is immobilized and five screws are placed in the mastoid cortex, pre-operative imaging is performed. The images are reconstructed into three dimensions using software. Using the 3D image, an ideal trajectory to the round window is planned (Fig. 6.1) [4, 7]. The second phase is accessing the middle ear. This phase requires careful intra-operative monitoring using imaging with a mobile cone-beam CT, and facial nerve monitoring. The HEARO-robotic system performs the drilling (Fig. 6.2) in three stages. The first stage is drilling from the cortex of the mastoid part of the temporal bone to 3 mm before the facial recess. A rod is then placed in the drilling hole followed by imaging. This stage is necessary to assess the safety margins and the executed trajectory. When a safe trajectory has been guaranteed, the second stage follows: further drilling through the facial recess in smaller steps of 0.5 mm, with facial nerve monitoring between successive steps. The third stage is the fastest part of the drilling process and achieves complete middle ear access (Fig. 6.3) [4]. The third and final phase of the HEARO-procedure is to attain inner ear access or milling of the canonus (Fig. 6.4), the bony overhang of the round window [8] (Fig. 6.5). During canonostomy, the drilling depth is

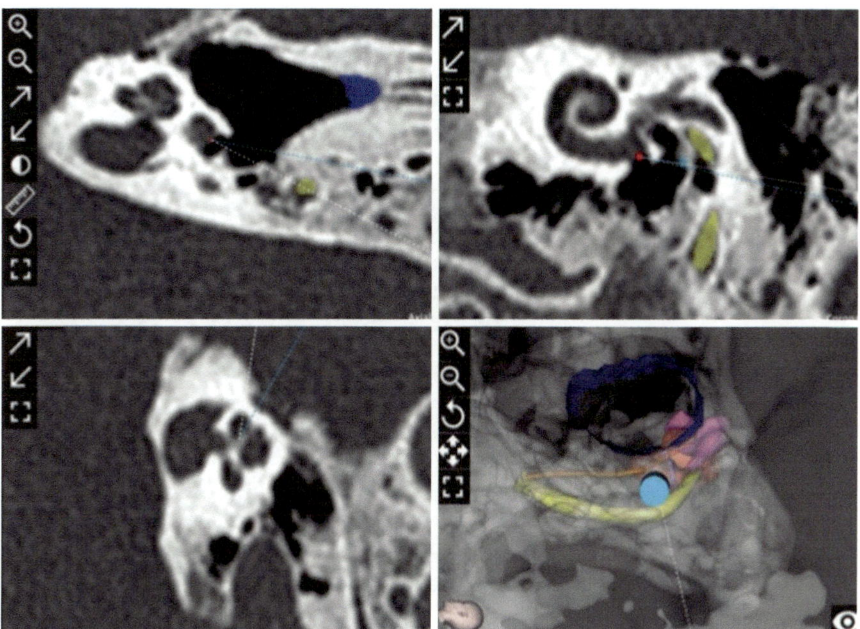

Fig. 6.1 A simulation of the optimal robotic drilling trajectory using planning software (OTOPLAN)

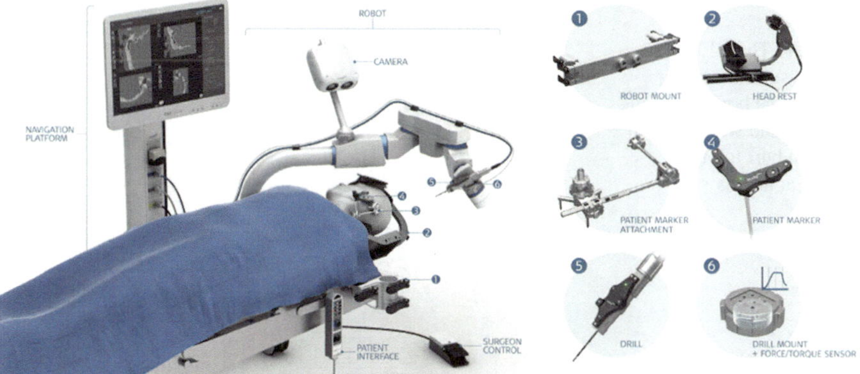

Fig. 6.2 The HEARO-robotic system

calculated from both imaging data and an intra-operative force-torque sensor (Fig. 6.6). After canonostomy, complete access to the inner ear has been achieved.

The surgeon then takes over manually. The electrode array of the cochlear implant device has to be placed correctly for the surgery to be deemed successful. From a transmeatal view, the insertion of the electrode array can be visualized by microscope or endoscope. After careful insertion through the drilling hole in the scala tympani of the cochlea, the surgeon fixates the implant and closes the wound

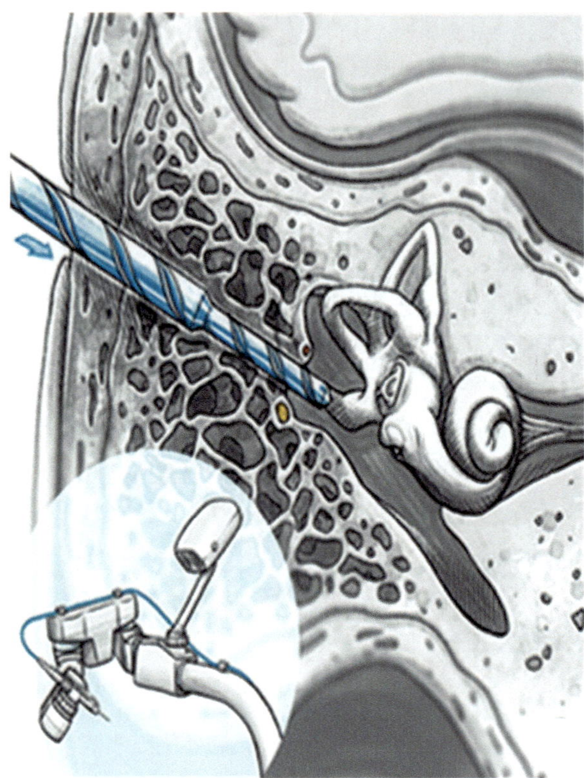

Fig. 6.3 The HEARO-robotic system drilling through the mastoid with a 1.8-mm drill to obtain middle ear access

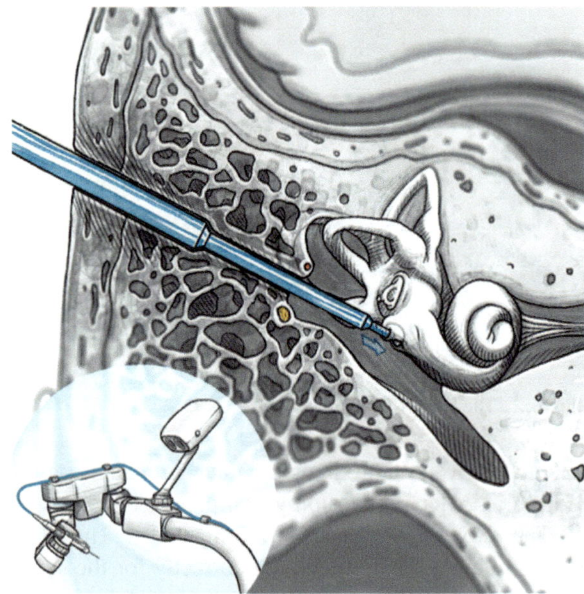

Fig. 6.4 The HEARO-robotic system milling through the bony overhang of the round window with a 1-mm burr to obtain inner ear access

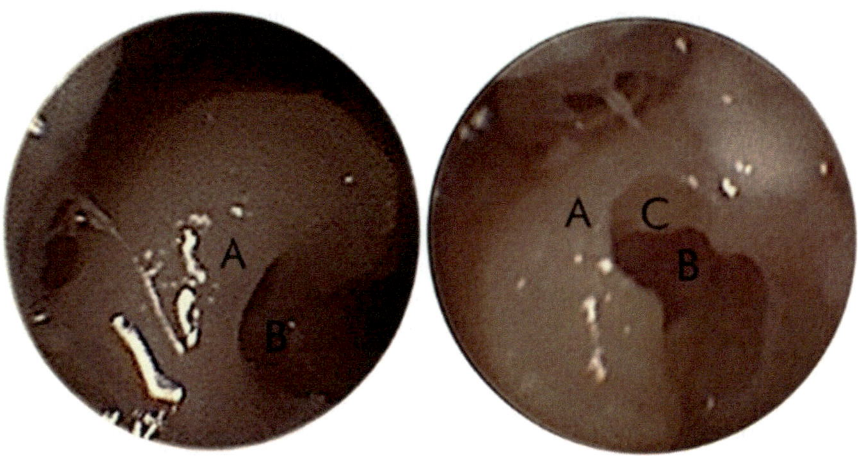

Fig. 6.5 An endoscopic view of the canonus (**a**), the round window (**b**) and a partial canonectomy (**c**)

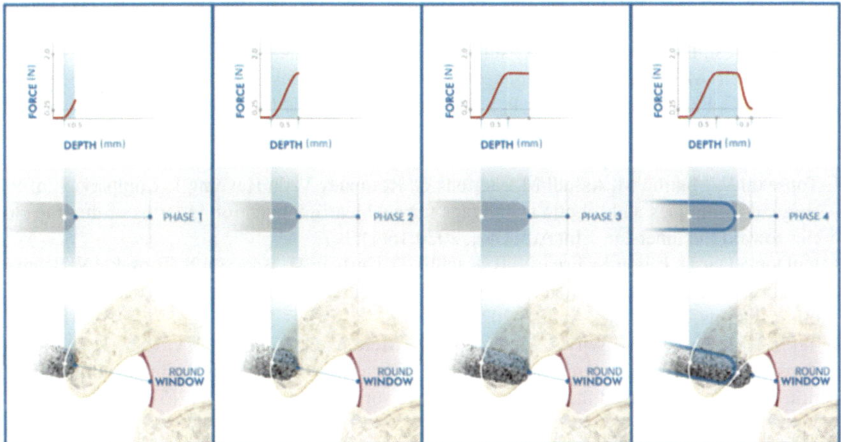

Fig. 6.6 A step-by-step illustration of inner ear access during the HEARO-procedure. The drill position is estimated using both an intra-operative force-torque sensor and pre-operative imaging

as in conventional cochlear implantation surgery. After surgery, post-operative imaging and electrophysiological tests are used to determine whether the placement of the electrode is correct [4, 9].

6.3 Conclusion and Future Perspectives

Robotically assisted cochlear implantation surgery is a minimally invasive way of performing autonomous inner ear access. Careful pre- and intra-operative planning makes atraumatic insertion of the electrode array possible, potentially providing better results than conventional surgery and also reducing operative and post-operative recovery times. The HEARO-procedure is still not a fully autonomous method of cochlear implantation surgery because autonomous electrode array insertion is not yet possible. Further studies are expected to make the procedure more efficient and safer.

References

1. Mertens G, Brandt A, Boudewyns A, Cochet E, Govaerts P, Lammers M, Topsakal V, Heyning P, Vanderveken O, Rompaey V. More than a quarter century of cochlear implantations: a retrospective study on 1161 implantations at the Antwerp University Hospital. B-ENT. 2021;17(3):155–63.
2. Topsakal V, Heuninck E, Matulic M, Tekin A, Mertens G, Van Rompaey V, Galeazzi P, Zoka-Assadi M, van de Heyning P. First study in men evaluating a surgical robotic tool providing autonomous inner ear access for Cochlear implantation. Front Neurol. 2022;13
3. Brown, C., Geers, A., Herrmann, B., Kirk, K., Tomblin, B. and Waltzman, S., 2004. Cochlear implants.
4. House W. Preface. Ann Otol Rhinol Laryngol. 1976;85(3_suppl):i–i.
5. Majdani O, Rau T, Baron S, Eilers H, Baier C, Heimann B, Ortmaier T, Bartling S, Lenarz T, Leinung M. A robot-guided minimally invasive approach for cochlear implant surgery: preliminary results of a temporal bone study. Int J Comput Assist Radiol Surg. 2009;4(5):475–86.
6. Caversaccio M, Gavaghan K, Wimmer W, Williamson T, Ansò J, Mantokoudis G, Gerber N, Rathgeb C, Feldmann A, Wagner F, Scheidegger O, Kompis M, Weisstanner C, Zoka-Assadi M, Roesler K, Anschuetz L, Huth M, Weber S. Robotic cochlear implantation: surgical procedure and first clinical experience. Acta Otolaryngol. 2017;137(4):447–54.
7. Topsakal V, Matulic M, Assadi M, Mertens G, Rompaey V, de Heyning P. Comparison of the surgical techniques and robotic techniques for cochlear implantation in terms of the trajectories toward the inner ear. J Int Adv Otol. 2020;16(1):3–7.
8. tenDonkelaar H, Elliott K, Fritzsch B, Kachlik D, Carlson M, Isaacson B, Topsakal V, Broman J, Tubbs S, Baud R. An updated terminology for the internal ear with combined anatomical and clinical terms. J Phonetics Audiol. 2022;6(2)
9. Tekin AM, Matulic M, Wuyts W, Assadi MZ, Mertens G, Rompaey VV, Li Y, Heyning PV, Topsakal V. A new pathogenic variant in POU3F4 causing deafness due to an incomplete partition of the cochlea paved the way for innovative surgery. Genes. 2021;12(5):613.

Robotics for Approaches to the Lateral Skull Base

7

Joachim Oertel and Jason Degiannis

7.1 Introduction

This chapter addresses the application of robotics in surgery of the lateral skull base. So far, very few data are available, so much of the chapter will be a theoretical evaluation of the pros and cons of robotics in the main approaches to the lateral skull base.

Historically, the first robotic-assisted procedure in neurosurgery was performed in 1985; it was a brain biopsy. Subsequently, robotic-assisted surgery was applied in many other aspects of neurosurgical practice, initially limited to intracranial and gradually expanding to spinal procedures [1]. Robots, not suffering from fatigue and tremor, improved the accuracy of stereotactic neurosurgical procedures by holding the surgical tools along the line produced by one or more pre-planned trajectories.

Over the following years, the number of publications slowly but continually increased. Nowadays, robot-assisted neurosurgery is used in treating several conditions.

Robotics is considered most helpful for *Stereoelectroencephalography* (SEEG) [2], in which electroencephalographic signals are recorded via deep electrodes. The accurate insertion and placement of the electrodes require "mapping" involving several trajectories, which can be significantly facilitated by a robot.

Additionally, in epilepsy surgery, *Radiofrequency Thermocoagulation* (RF-THC) and *Laser Interstitial Thermal Therapy* (LiTT) can be applied if small volumes of surrounding brain tissue need to be ablated in reoperations [3].

J. Oertel (✉) · J. Degiannis
Klinik für Neurochirurgie, Universitätsklinikum des Saarlandes, Medizinische Fakultät, Universität des Saarlandes, Homburg, Germany
e-mail: Joachim.Oertel@uks.eu; Jason.Degiannis@uks.eu

M. M. Al-Salihi et al. (eds.), *Robotics in Skull-Base Surgery*,
https://doi.org/10.1007/978-3-031-38376-2_7

Chronic high-frequency *Deep Brain Stimulation* (DBS) results in ablation of selected areas of functional brain parenchyma. This improves treatment results in motor disorders, the most common indication being Parkinson's disease. Robot-assisted insertion of stimulating electrodes into the subthalamic nucleus and the subsequent deep brain stimulation improves not only the tremor but also the rigidity and the bradykinetic symptoms and signs associated with the disorder [1, 4, 5].

Robotic assistance in taking biopsies is superior to any other method, as it enhances the surgeon's skills with accuracy and mechanical stability. It enables the surgeon to obtain multi-bite biopsies of the lesion and the surrounding tissue, enabling the correct histological diagnosis to be made through the full extent of the tumor [1].

Robotic neuro-endoscopy [6] has been applied in the resection of hypothalamic hamartomas and has also been used to relieve obstructive hydrocephalus and fenestration of cerebral cysts in pediatric patients. It has recently been used to treat hemispheric epilepsy by performing hemispherectomy [1].

There is a gradual increase in the number of indications for robot-assisted spinal surgery. A robot can guide the surgeon to deep anatomical areas through a narrow corridor while avoiding vital anatomical structures. At present, the most widely used procedures are pedicle-screw placement and anterior lumbar interbody fusion (ALIF).

During earlier robotic applications, the position of the microscope or the endoscope was the focus [7, 8], but nowadays true robotic surgery with micromanipulators and joysticks receives increasing emphasis. However, only in stereotactic functional applications can robotics really be considered to have been incorporated to a limited degree into daily clinical routine [9, 10].

The lateral skull base is a particularly challenging area for the neurosurgeon. Not only are the lower cranial nerves involved in this area but also the two carotid arteries and vertebral arteries as well as the draining veins. Additionally, many different approaches are available with distinct pros and cons depending on objective criteria and the subjective opinion of the performing surgeon.

In the following, the authors present the peculiarities of standard approaches to the lateral skull base such as the pterional and frontolateral and the retromastoid and far lateral approaches.

7.2 Pterional and Frontolateral Approaches to the Lateral Anterior and Middle Cranial Fossae

Named after the pterion, which is the junction of four bones—the temporal, frontal, parietal, and the sphenoid (greater wing)—the pterional approach is one of the five most important approaches to the lateral skull base. It is especially useful for lesions in the lateral aspect of the skull base, such as subfrontal, temporal, parasellar, tentorial, and midline lesions. It is the gold standard for microsurgical management of cerebral aneurysms involving the anterior part of the circle of Willis [11, 12]. The patient is placed in supine position and the head is slightly extended and rotated to

30–60 degrees, depending on the anatomical site of the lesion, allowing the zygoma to be the highest point. Owing to gravity, the frontal lobe then falls away from the anterior cranial fossa, facilitating access to the lesion. Slight lateral flexion of the cervical spine to the contralateral side makes the Sylvian fissure lie vertically in relation to the surgeon [13].

The authors apply this approach mainly in surgery for lesions around the internal carotid artery, the cavernous sinus, and the anterior clinoid process. The approach is presented in detail in Fig. 7.1.

The frontolateral approach is distinguished from the pterional approach by its more medial extension. The Sylvian fissure is only partially exposed. It allows the skull to be accessed via the anterior cranial fossa and to some degree the middle cranial fossa. It is often used for the resection of olfactory groove meningiomas and for subfrontal, parasellar, and tentorial lesions [12].

Preparation for the frontolateral approach shares many similarities with the pterional approach. However, since it is more frontal and more medial, the head is usually less rotated and the route is subfrontal with the frontal lobe mainly elevated, in contrast to the pterional approach, which has a rather transfissural trajectory. The authors apply this approach mainly for surgery of lesions around the internal carotid artery, the cavernous sinus, and the anterior clinoid process. It is their preferred approach because it does not require drilling most of the sphenoid wing, and only minimal dissection of the Sylvian fissure is needed. Thus, they prefer the

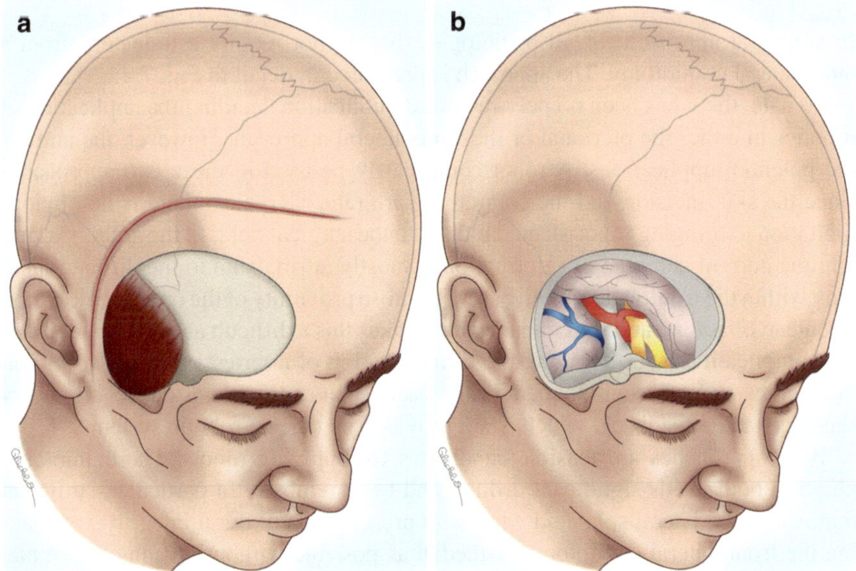

Fig. 7.1 Pterional approach (Courtesy of Laura Glucklich). (**a**) Schematic drawing of skin incision and craniotomy size in relation to pterion and temporalis muscle. (**b**) Schematic drawing of intraoperative view of carotid artery with junction of anterior and middle cerebral arteries and optic nerve. Please note the easy approach to the Sylvian fissure

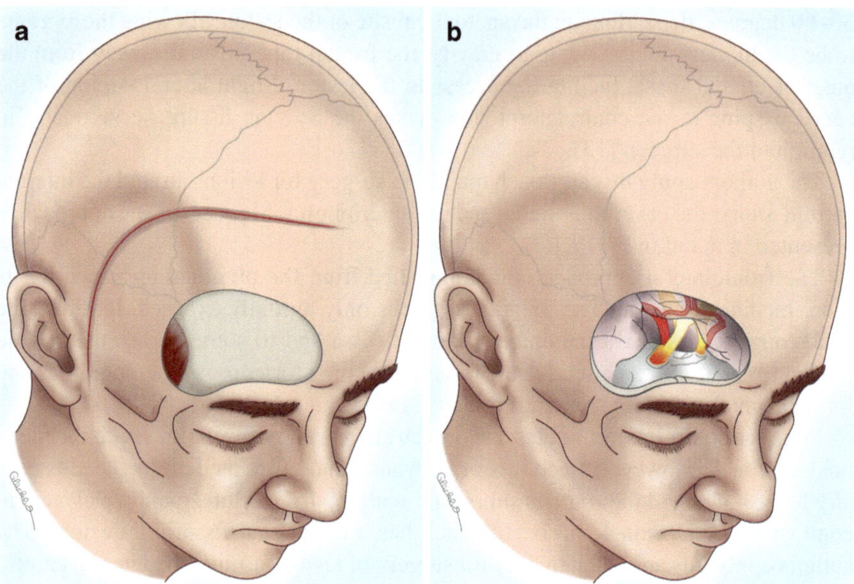

Fig. 7.2 Frontolateral approach (Courtesy of Laura Glucklich). (**a**) Schematic drawing of skin incision and craniotomy size in relation to pterion and temporalis muscle. (**b**) Schematic drawing of intraoperative view of carotid artery with junction of anterior and middle cerebral arteries and optic nerve. Please note the easy approach to the optic nerves and optic chiasm

frontolateral approach for all pathologies that do not require a trajectory from a more lateral craniotomy. The approach is presented in detail in Fig. 7.2.

To date, there has been no peer-reviewed publication detailing the application of robotics in either the pterional or the frontolateral approach. However, the authors see potential applications. A robot could easily be used in these two approaches since the skin incision and the craniotomy are rather large, so there is no obvious limitation to bringing robot-steered tools into the surgical field. In the authors' opinion, the current shortage of information is mostly attributable to the difficult anatomy within the frontolateral skull base. The close proximity of the optic, oculomotor, trochlear, olfactory, and trigeminal nerves makes this a difficult area with a high risk for complications. Furthermore, the differentiation of arteries and veins from cranial nerves and adjacent eloquent brain tissue such as the brainstem requires very sensitive tactile feedback, which is not provided by current robotic systems.

Both approaches are feasible candidates for applying robots. The craniotomy phase in both needs significant drilling and bone removal. In particular, sufficient removal of the lateral sphenoid wing with preservation of dural integrity and making the frontolateral craniotomy as medial as possible without opening the frontal sinus, appear well suited to robotic-controlled craniotomy. In the intracranial phase, very delicate structures with different tissue resistances such as arteries, veins, and cranial nerves—as discussed above—make these approaches difficult for robotics, although the expected high accuracy of a robot could lower the operative risk significantly. Therefore, the authors are convinced that robotics will become valuable for treating lesions of the anterior and middle fossa skull base via pterional and frontolateral craniotomy. However, more experience is needed before such different surgeries can be done with the aid of robotics.

7.3 Retrosigmoid (Lateral Suboccipital) and Far Lateral Approaches to the Lateral Posterior Fossa

The retrosigmoid approach is the "bread and butter" approach for the lateral posterior cranial fossa in neurosurgery. It is also one of the five most important approaches, comparable in importance to the pterional approach to the anterior and middle cranial fossa. It is especially useful for lesions in the cerebellopontine angle, at the subtentorial lateral petrous bone, and in the lateral foramen magnum. It is the gold standard for a microsurgical approach to many meningiomas, schwannomas, chordomas, and metastases in this region. The key step is to identify the asterion, the junction of the lambdoid, occipitomastoid, and parietomastoid sutures. Directly beneath these sutures run the transverse and sigmoid sinuses, which frequently have to be exposed; particular care is needed to avoid injuries to these structures.

For the approach, the patient is placed in a prone, lateral, or semi-sitting position. The authors prefer the semi-sitting position for various reasons; however, the individual preferences of surgeons vary widely. In the semi-sitting position (please also refer to reference 13) the head is slightly elevated, inclined toward the sternum and rotated 30–45° toward the lesion. Intraoperative transesophageal echocardiography is very helpful for early detection of air embolism. To reduce the risk of air embolism further, the patient's legs should be elevated, and the blood should be pooled around the chest. Therefore, the table is usually flexed to facilitate venous return.

After shaving, skin disinfection and sterile draping, the mastoid tip is located. In difficult anatomical situations, neuronavigation can be used. The site of the skin incision depends on the lesion. The greater the need to see inside the internal acoustic meatus, the more medial the skin incision should be. As a rule of thumb, the skin incision is made 3 cm behind the ear, extending from the upper ear level down to the mastoid tip. Dissection of the muscles follows, with care to avoid injury to the lesser and greater occipital nerves and occipital artery, although this is frequently not possible. Then the skull sutures and the anatomical orientation points are identified: Asterion, lambdoid suture, parietomastoid suture, occipitomastoid suture. The transverse and sigmoid sinuses are then located. Then the craniotomy is performed close to the sinus with an osteoplastic followed by an osteoclastic technique, finally exposing these veins. The osteoclastic technique includes partial mastoidectomy for exposure to the sigmoid sinus.

The authors apply this approach mainly in surgery for lesions around the cerebellopontine angle and the subtentorial lateral petrous part of the temporal bone, and lesions anterolateral to the foramen magnum. It is also the preferred approach for many vascular lesions of the posterior fossa. It is presented in detail in Fig. 7.3.

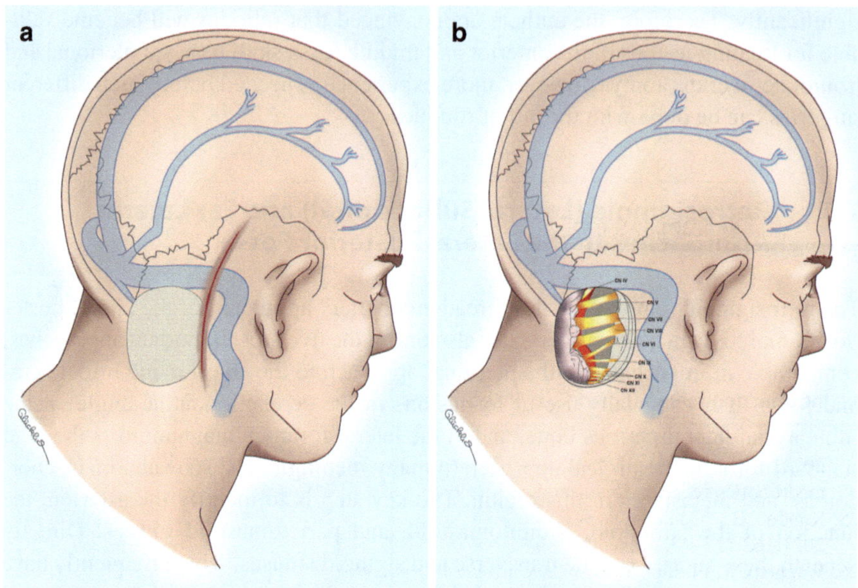

Fig. 7.3 Retrosigmoid approach (Courtesy of Laura Glucklich). (**a**) Schematic drawing of skin incision and craniotomy size in relation to the asterion and both sigmoid and transverse sinuses. (**b**) Schematic drawing of intraoperative view of the cerebellopontine angle with cranial nerves IV through XII and basilar and vertebral arteries

The far lateral approach is essentially an extension of a lateral suboccipital approach with an opening of the foramen magnum. There are many different extensions depending on which site of surgery is desired. It has therefore been dubbed the "Far lateral enough approach," as additional removal of bony components such as the condylar fossa, the occipital condyle, and the jugular tubercle is required. Following extensive removals of the condyles, dorsal stabilization should be ensured to avoid biomechanical instability of the atlantooccipital joint [13, 14].

This approach is used for access to lesions of the anterior and anterolateral clivus, the brainstem, the craniovertebral junction, and the upper spine. It is presented in detail in Fig. 7.4.

No detailed application of robotics in these infratentorial approaches has been described to date. As in the approaches to the anterior and middle cranial fossa, a robot could easily be used in these two approaches since the skin incision and the craniotomy are rather large, so there is no obvious limitation to bringing robot-steered tools into the surgical field. However, in the retrosigmoid approach, the delicate anatomy in the cerebellopontine angle makes it difficult to deploy a robot. Because of the close proximity of cranial nerves III through XII in conjunction with the vertebral and basilar arteries, this area has a high risk for intraoperative complications. Furthermore, differentiating arteries and veins from cranial nerves and adjacent eloquent brain tissue such as the brain stem requires very sensitive tactile feedback, which is not provided by current robotic systems. The application could

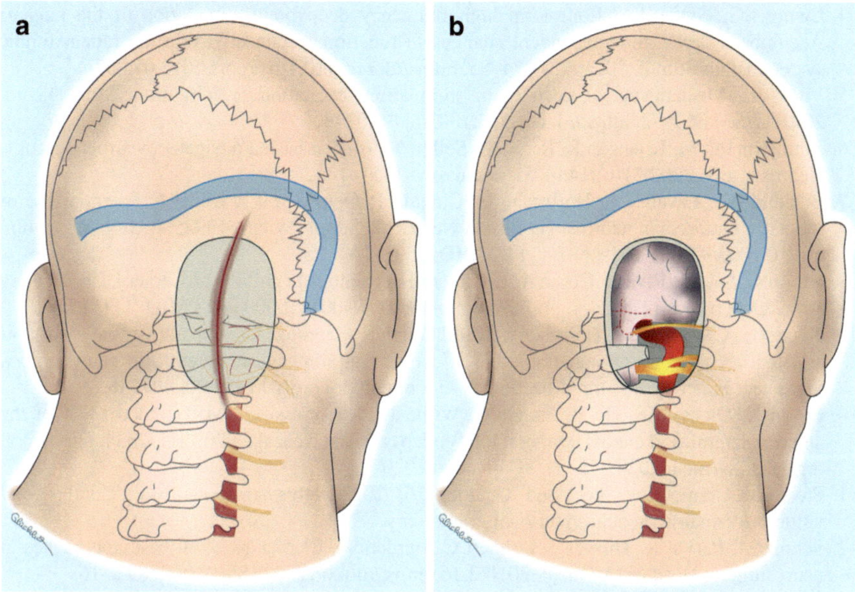

Fig. 7.4 Far lateral approach (Courtesy of Laura Glucklich). (**a**) Schematic drawing of skin incision and craniotomy size in relation to the foramen magnum, C1, and extracranial vertebral artery. (**b**) Schematic drawing of intraoperative view of the craniovertebral junction via a far lateral approach

be more feasible in the far lateral approach; but since this approach is quite rare, it is not necessarily the first choice procedure for starting robotic applications.

In summary, both approaches are feasible candidates for applying a robot. The craniotomy phase in both requires significant drilling and bone removal, as in pterional and frontolateral craniotomy. In particular, sufficient removal of the suboccipital bone with preservation of the sinus and dural integrity could be an interesting first application of a robot in these approaches. The authors are convinced that robotics will become valuable in these lateral posterior fossa approaches in the future. However, more experience is needed before such different surgeries can be performed with the aid of robotics.

References

1. Martínez JA, González CF. Robotics in neurosurgery: principles and practice. Springer Nature; 2022.
2. Iida K, Otsubo H. Stereoelectroencephalography: indication and efficacy. Neurol Med Chir. 2017;57(8):375–85. https://doi.org/10.2176/nmc.ra.2017-0008.
3. Wang Y-C, Cheng M-Y, Hung P-C, Kuo C-Y, Hsieh H-Y, Lin K-L, Po-Hsun T, et al. Robot-assisted radiofrequency ablation combined with thermodynamic simulation for epilepsy reoperations. J Clin Med. 2022;11(16):4804. https://doi.org/10.3390/jcm11164804.

4. Ewing SG, Grace AA. Long-term high frequency deep brain stimulation of the nucleus Accumbens drives time-dependent changes in functional connectivity in the rodent limbic system. Brain Stimul. 2013;6(3):274–85. https://doi.org/10.1016/j.brs.2012.07.007.
5. Vitek JL. Mechanisms of deep brain stimulation: excitation or inhibition. Mov Disord. 2002;17(S3):S69–72. https://doi.org/10.1002/mds.10144.
6. Zimmermann M, Krishnan R, Raabe A, Seifert V. Robot-assisted navigated Neuroendoscopy. Neurosurgery. 2002;51(6):1446–51. discussion 1451–1452
7. Benabid AL, Lavallee S, Hoffmann D, Cinquin P, Demongeot J, Danel F. Potential use of robots in endoscopic neurosurgery. Acta Neurochir Suppl (Wien). 1992;54:93–7. https://doi.org/10.1007/978-3-7091-6687-1_14. PMID: 1595416
8. Giorgi C, Sala R, Riva D, Cossu A, Eisenberg H. Robotics in child neurosurgery. Childs Nerv Syst. 2000;16(10–11):832–4. https://doi.org/10.1007/s003810000394. PMID: 11151738
9. Neudorfer C, Hunsche S, Hellmich M, El Majdoub F, Maarouf M. Comparative study of robot-assisted versus conventional frame-based deep brain stimulation stereotactic neurosurgery. Stereotact Funct Neurosurg. 2018;96:327–34. https://doi.org/10.1159/000494736.
10. Gupta K, Dickey AS, Hu R, Faught E, Willie JT. Robot-assisted MRI-guided LITT of the anterior, lateral, and medial temporal lobe epilepsy. Front Neurol. 2020;11:572334. https://doi.org/10.3389/fneur.2020.572334. eCollection 2020
11. Pterional Craniotomy. Accessed October 16, 2022. https://www.neurosurgicalatlas.com/volumes/cranial-approaches/pterional-craniotomy
12. Scholz M, Parvin R, Thissen J, Löhnert C, Harders A, Blaeser K. Skull base approaches in neurosurgery. Head Neck Oncol. 2010;2:16. https://doi.org/10.1186/1758-3284-2-16.
13. Raabe A, Meyer B, Schaller K, Vajkoczy P, Peter A, editors. The Craniotomy Atlas. Winkler, New York: Thieme; 2019. p. 112–217.
14. Far-Lateral and Extreme Lateral Approaches. Accessed October 16, 2022. https://www.neurosurgicalatlas.com/volumes/operative-neuroanatomy/infratentorial-operative-anatomy/far-lateral-and-extreme-lateral-approaches

Robotics in Radiosurgery

8

Shawn S. Rai, Lawrence S. Chin, Harish Babu, and Mohammed Maan Al-Salihi

8.1 Gamma Knife

Gamma Knife™ (Elekta) radiosurgery was developed by Leksell and Larsson in 1967. The gamma rays emitted from the apparatus are photon beams produced by radioactive decay that ionize the irradiated tissue (Fig. 8.1). Traditionally, computed tomography (CT) or magnetic resonance imaging (MRI) scans are obtained after the patient is positioned within a Leksell fixed headframe. Proprietary software is then used by the treatment team to select the target after a fixed three-dimensional relationship is composed between target and frame. A hemispheric array of 192 cobalt-60 collimators allows the gamma-ray beams to be focused accurately on the lesion at the center of their intersection while minimizing unwanted irradiation of surrounding tissue. The circular array of 192 beams allows treatment planning to be adapted significantly. When the targeted lesion is not spherical but eccentrically shaped, multiple spherical treatments can be planned to treat it. The updated Gamma Knife system (Perfexion™) now includes a hemispheric collimator array in the main housing, precluding the need for the patient to wear a helmet as in previous versions (Gamma Knife C™). Gamma Knife radiosurgery is limited in that it is only used in cranial and upper cervical lesions because frame-based stereotaxis on a rigid skull is required. Also, treatments can only be given in a single session, precluding dose fractionation over multiple appointments [5–8].

S. S. Rai
Department of Neurosurgery, Emory University School of Medicine, Atlanta, GA, USA

L. S. Chin · H. Babu (✉)
Department of Neurosurgery, SUNY Upstate Medical University, Syracuse, NY, USA
e-mail: BabuH@upstate.edu

M. M. Al-Salihi
Department of Neurological Surgery, School of Medicine and Public Health, University of Wisconsin, Madison, WI, USA

M. M. Al-Salihi et al. (eds.), *Robotics in Skull-Base Surgery*, https://doi.org/10.1007/978-3-031-38376-2_8

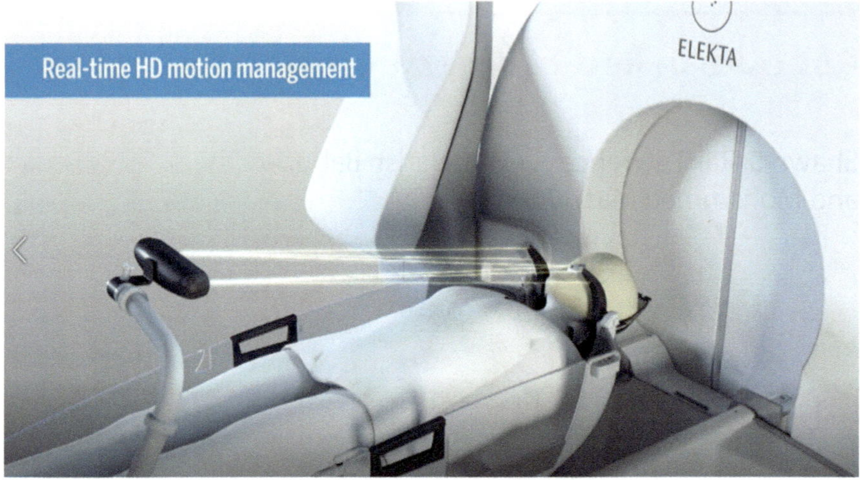

Fig. 8.1 Real-time high-definition motion management system. Yamaguchi H (January 03, 2022) Gamma Knife Radiosurgery with Mask Fixation Under General Anesthesia for Pediatric Patients. Cureus 14(1): e20905. doi:10.7759/cureus.20905

8.2 Robotics in Gamma Knife

Advances in robotics have also allowed Gamma Knife radiosurgery to be automated by allowing a robot to position the Leksell frame, enabling each radiation dose to be focused on the lesion [3]. Automating a significant portion of the Gamma Knife treatment process minimizes the need for manual input for patient positioning by the treatment team and decreases treatment time.

Robotics has also allowed a frameless-based Gamma Knife system to be developed (Gamma Knife Icon™). The updated frameless-based Gamma Knife system uses a polystyrene cushion in which the patient's head is fixed. An oven heated, three-point thermoplastic mask is then used to achieve relative immobilization of the patient's head. Gamma Knife Icon™ uses infrared stereoscopic cameras on a movable arm attached to the patient's couch. Reference markers within the patient's custom-fit mask and an adhesive sticker placed on the patient's nose are used to determine patient movement in relation to a preset threshold. If the threshold is breached, the treatment is automatically paused. The robotic-controlled movement of the treatment couch, conformal therapy from the Gamma Knife Icon™ housing, and the frameless-based head immobilization allow for significant improvement in patient comfort and efficiency as there is no need for frame placement. Non-rigid immobilization with the aforementioned stereotactic mask is best used for patients who are relaxed and able to remain relatively motionless for a prolonged period. Frameless-based Gamma Knife radiosurgery also allows for the fractionation of treatment, allowing higher combined total doses to be delivered to the lesion over multiple sessions [7, 8] (Fig. 8.2).

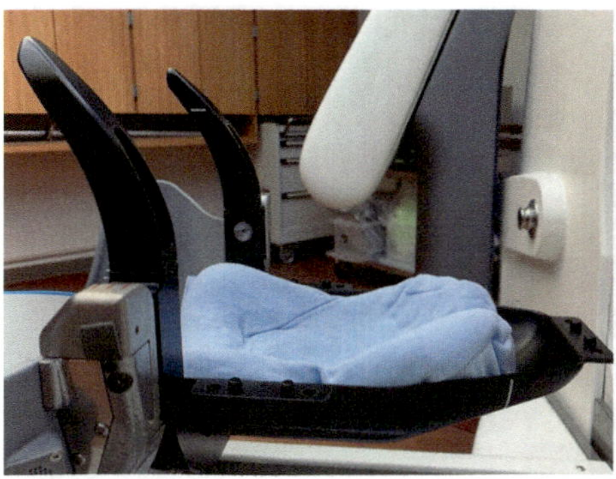
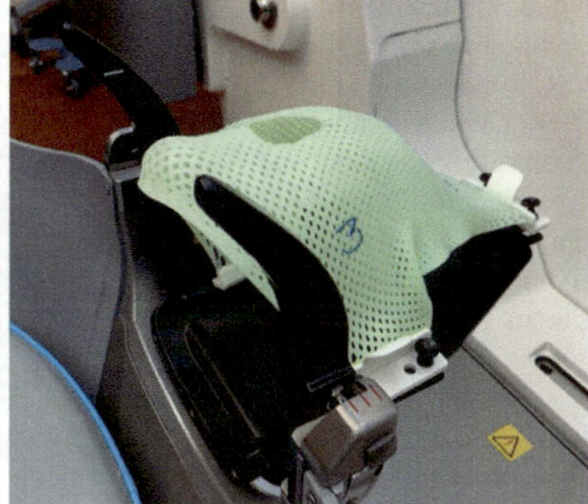

Fig. 8.2 Mask adapter for Gamma Knife Icon. Mendel J T, Schroeder S, Plitt A, et al. (March 19, 2021) Expanded Radiosurgery Capabilities Utilizing Gamma Knife Icon™. Cureus 13(3): e13998. doi:10.7759/cureus.13998

Frame-based Gamma Knife radiosurgery is also limited in treating several metastatic lesions in a single session owing to total treatment time and potential dose overlap between multiple treatment plans for various targets [9]. Frameless-based Gamma Knife radiosurgery allows treatments for multiple lesions to be distributed over several sessions, lowering the risks of radiation necrosis, edema, and treatment toxicity [7].

8.3 Linear Accelerator

The Linac system uses X-rays emitted from a linear accelerator. These photon beams are produced by electron acceleration. The accelerator is rotated around the patient in a circular motion allowing the treatment team to change the delivery angle aimed at the specified lesion. The patient's position on the couch can also be changed to allow the beam delivery angles to be customized further. The limitation of the Linac treatment system is that it works in a two-dimensional space. Owing to this limitation, the targeted lesion is most amendable to treatment when near osseous structures, such as brain lesions close to the spinal apparatus [4, 6, 10].

8.4 Robotic Linear Accelerator (CyberKnife)

The CyberKnife (Accuray™) system is like the isocentric Linac system in that it also uses a linear accelerator as a radiation source. It uses a robot to move the radiation source to various points to deliver radiation doses from various angles while creating a three-dimensional treatment paradigm (Fig. 8.3). The CyberKnife system uses a robot with six degrees of freedom of movement with a mounted linear accelerator to direct the photon beam onto the targeted lesion. Treatment planning is similar to the Gamma Knife system. Identification of the targeted lesion and surrounding critical structures is completed using propriety software and a high-quality pre-treatment CT. The proprietary software then uses a number of points on a virtual

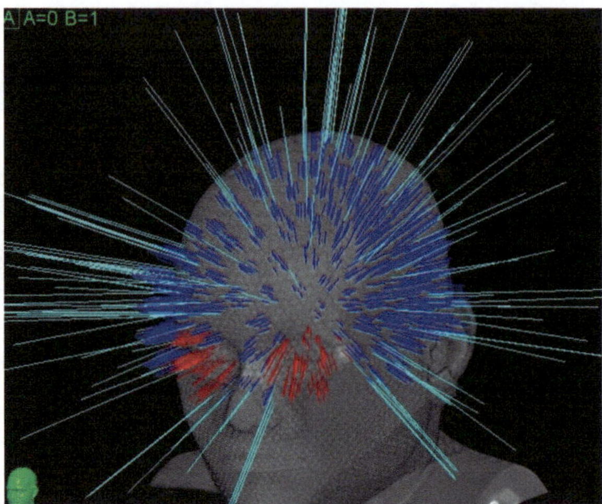

Fig. 8.3 Treatment planning shown on T1W MR. Romanelli P (July 12, 2018) CyberKnife® Radiosurgery as First-line Treatment for Catastrophic Epilepsy Caused by Hypothalamic Hamartoma. Cureus 10(7): e2968. doi:10.7759/cureus.2968

treatment sphere to determine beam directions and dosage to achieve conformity within the planned treatment target [1, 8, 11].

The novel feature of the CyberKnife system compared to previous versions of Linac systems is the continuous image-guided loop. Two X-ray cameras are used to assess patient positioning continuously relative to the planned treatment. The X-rays are compared to the pre-treatment CT, and the robotic treatment beam positions are automatically corrected as the patient's position changes. This process continues throughout the treatment process. Because of this design, the CyberKnife system has several advantages. Owing to the ability to use frameless-based treatment and the open design of the system, the CyberKnife can treat the entire body of the patient rather than be limited to the head and upper cervical region, as with the Gamma Knife system (Fig. 8.4). Also, the real-time optimization of treatment trajectories based on patient positioning allows lesions to be targeted within anatomical locations that are more susceptible to patient movement, e.g., lesions within the lung that move with each respiration. The ability to treat other organ systems makes the CyberKnife system attractive for healthcare systems. The continuous tracking of the patient's position during treatment also allows for frameless-based treatment, increasing patient comfort and time efficiency. Hypofractionated doses over multiple sessions can also be given with the CyberKnife system, allowing for lower toxicity while maintaining a high cumulative treatment dose. The accuracy of the robotic system has also improved and is similar to that of the well-established historical gold standard of Gamma Knife frame-based systems [1, 12–15].

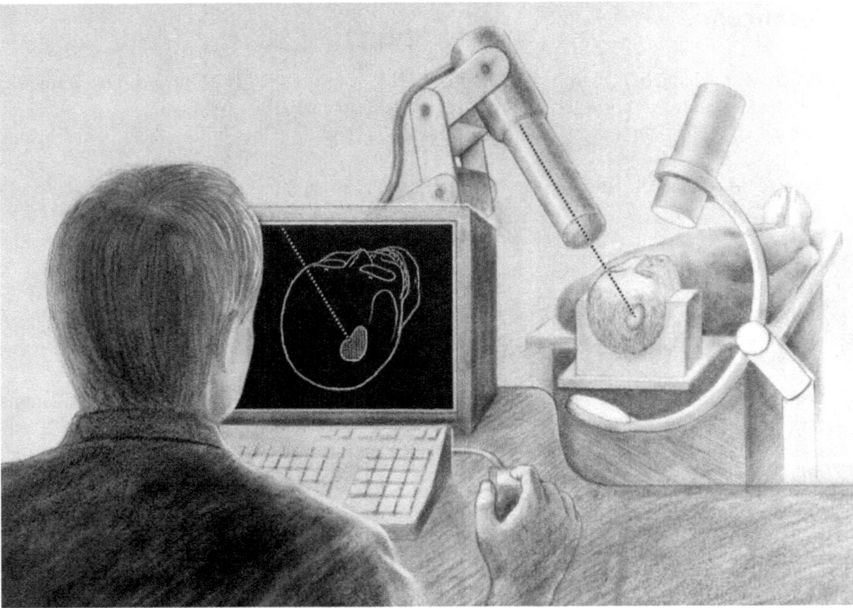

Fig. 8.4 Made in 1988 this image depicts the initial concepts of the frameless radiosurgical technology which would eventually become the CyberKnife. Adler J R. (September 15, 2009) Accuray, Inc.: A Neurosurgical Business Case Study. Cureus 1(9): e1. doi:10.7759/cureus.1

8.5 Conclusion

Robotics has made significant contributions to radiosurgery. Radiosurgery has traditionally been limited to frame-based technologies such as Gamma Knife and stereotactic linear accelerators. New iterations of the Gamma Knife system (Icon™) and the linear accelerator (CyberKnife™) using precision robotics have allowed for frameless-based radiosurgery. Frameless techniques improve patient comfort and offer real-time correction of patient movement during treatment while maintaining accuracy. Robotics has also led to a significant increase in the efficiency of treatment of multiple lesions, the ability to offer hypo-fractionated treatment over multiple sessions, and the capacity to treat extracranial pathologies. Robotics will increasingly allow for radiosurgical treatment of diseases within the spine. Also, robotics makes the treatment of several intracranial metastatic lesions more practical. Future development of robots with increased degrees of freedom, increased computing power, and improved software will allow for more efficient and accurate treatment while minimizing patient morbidity.

References

1. Adler JR Jr, Chang SD, Murphy MJ, Doty J, Geis P, Hancock SL. The Cyberknife: a frameless robotic system for radiosurgery. Stereotact Funct Neurosurg. 1997;69:124–8.
2. Leksell L. The stereotaxic method and radiosurgery of the brain. Acta Chir Scand. 1951;102:316–9.
3. Jayarao M, Chin LS. Robotics and its applications in stereotactic radiosurgery. Neurosurg Focus. 2007;23:E6.
4. Colombo F, Benedetti A, Pozza F, et al. External stereotactic irradiation by linear accelerator. Neurosurgery. 1985;16:154–60.
5. Ganz JC. Changing the gamma knife. Prog Brain Res. 2014;215:117–25.
6. Xing LTB, Schreibmann E, Yang Y, Li TF, Kim GY. Dosim eaOoi-grtM. 31:91–112. Jayarao M, Chin LS Robotics and its applications in stereotactic radiosurgery Neurosurgical focus 2007;23:E6.
7. Mendel JT, Schroeder S, Plitt A, et al. Expanded radiosurgery capabilities utilizing gamma knife icon™. Cureus. 2021;13:e13998.
8. Luan S, Swanson N, Chen Z, Ma L. Dynamic gamma knife radiosurgery. Phys Med Biol. 2009;54:1579–91.
9. Yamamoto M, Kawabe T, Sato Y, et al. Stereotactic radiosurgery for patients with multiple brain metastases: a case-matched study comparing treatment results for patients with 2-9 versus 10 or more tumors. J Neurosurg. 2014;121(Suppl):16–25.
10. Noh SY, Jeong K, Seo Y-c, et al. Development of a prototype robotic system for radiosurgery with upper hemispherical workspace. Journal of healthcare. Engineering. 2017;2017:4264356.
11. Adler JR Jr. The future of robotics in radiosurgery. Neurosurgery. 2013;72(Suppl 1):8–11.
12. Kresl JJ. St. Joseph's hospital and Barrow neurological institute stereotactic radiotherapy experience: comparison of gamma knife and CyberKnife. Nowotwory. J Oncol. 2006;56:125.
13. Levivier M, Gevaert T, Negretti L. Gamma knife, cyberknife, tomotherapy: gadgets or useful tools? Curr Opin Neurol. 2011;24:616–25.
14. Wowra B, Muacevic A, Tonn JC. CyberKnife radiosurgery for brain metastases. Prog Neurol Surg. 2012;25:201–9.
15. Chang SD, Main W, Martin DP, Gibbs IC, Heilbrun MP. An analysis of the accuracy of the CyberKnife: a robotic frameless stereotactic radiosurgical system. Neurosurgery. 2003;52:140–6. discussion 6–7

Robotics in Neurotology 9

Thomas Lenarz, Rolf Benedikt Salcher, and Samuel John

9.1 Surgical Procedures and Other Interventions in Neurotology

9.1.1 Challenges and Surgical Principles

Neurotology deals with diseases of hearing and balance which are originating from the temporal bone and its surrounding structures (Fig. 9.1). The temporal bone can be divided into distinct anatomical regions and is composed of the hardest bone of the human body and extremely delicate soft tissue structures, most of them on a (sub)millimeter scale. It houses the sensory organs of hearing and balance with the associated vestibulocochlear nerve, the external and middle ears, and the Eustachian tube. It is a major pathway for nerves and major vessels to and from the brain, such as the facial nerve, the lower cranial nerves, the carotid artery, and several dural venous sinuses. It is part of the middle and posterior cranial fossa in close contact with several parts of the brain including the temporal and occipital lobes, and the brain stem.

Surgical procedures in the temporal bone must follow specific principles to achieve the following goals: Removal of pathologies, i.e., benign or cancerous

T. Lenarz · R. B. Salcher
Department of Otorhinolaryngology, Head and Neck Surgery, Hannover Medical School, Hanover, Germany
e-mail: lenarz.thomas@mh-hannover.de; salcher.rolf@mh-hannover.de

S. John (✉)
Department of Otorhinolaryngology, Head and Neck Surgery, Hannover Medical School, Hanover, Germany

OtoJig GmbH, Hanover, Germany
e-mail: john.samuel@otojig.com

M. M. Al-Salihi et al. (eds.), *Robotics in Skull-Base Surgery*, https://doi.org/10.1007/978-3-031-38376-2_9

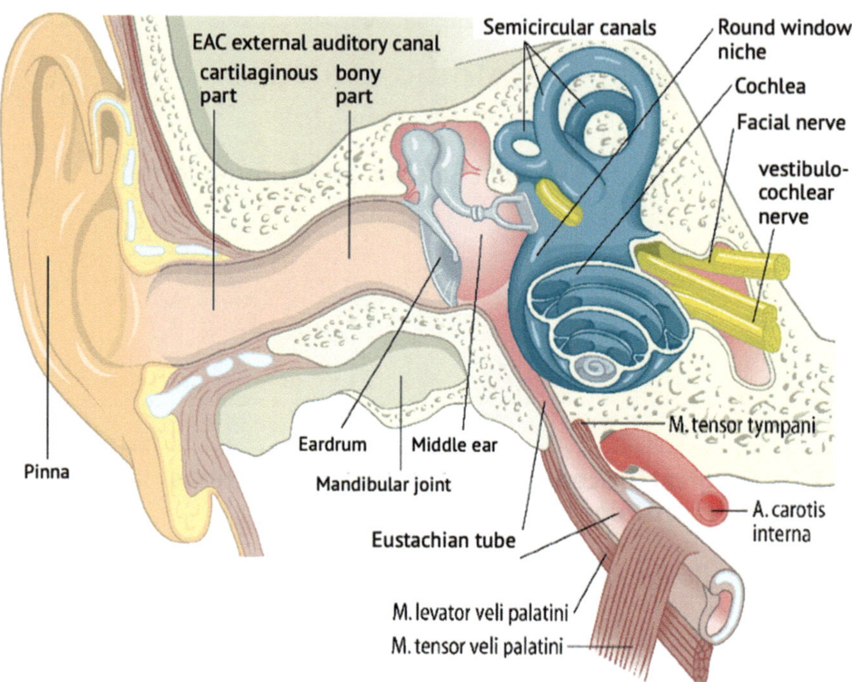

Fig. 9.1 Overview of the anatomy of the human temporal bone from the outer ear (pinna), to the middle ear with the ossicular chain, and the inner ear (cochlea) including the vestibule and semicircular canals

tumors, reconstruction of anatomical structures, for example, parts of the ossicular chain, and/or implantation to treat example hearing loss.

The surgeon must have a deep knowledge of the complex underlying anatomy and sophisticated manual skills to perform the surgical procedures on a microscopic scale and be able to identify and expose delicate structures with important functions within the bone. Some of the procedures must be performed without direct visual control, e.g., electrode insertion in cochlear implantation.

Over the last decades, important technological innovations were added to the toolbox of the neurotologist to improve both diagnostics and therapy. New treatments have become possible and opened new areas of patient management. Their integration into the workflow has become a challenging task and can be only performed by an interdisciplinary and well-trained team including otologists, neurosurgeons, audiologists, neuroradiologists, OR assistants, as well as technicians. The most important innovations are high-resolution digital microscopes including 3D imaging, miniaturized endoscopic imaging, (intraoperative) high-resolution cone beam computed tomography, high-resolution MRI, interventional neuroradiology with embolization and vascular stenting, optical or electromagnetic neuronavigation for intraoperative localization of anatomical structures, neuromonitoring of neural and sensory functions, ablation techniques including laser, piezoelectric, and ultrasound aspiration, as well as precision radiotherapy.

These innovations claim to improve the results of surgical procedures in neurotology toward less invasive, more targeted interventions with reduced functional impairment and less side effects as well as better functional outcome and quality of life.

The application and combination of these different technologies is still a huge challenge due to the limitation of available physical space in the operating theater, the additional time for setting up these devices, the different data formats, arranging all the separate displays, missing interconnections and a lack compatibilities among the systems. However, there are initiatives to standardize connectivity and interoperability of medical devices in the operating room [1].

9.2 Potential Advantages of Robotics in Neurotology

What are people expecting from robotics? Science fiction movies such as the sci-fi thriller "Transcendence" by Jack Paglen (Warner Bros. Motion Pictures) drive the expectation of fully autonomous, superhuman, AI-powered surgical robots that are minimally invasive with extreme speed and accuracy. From industrial manufacturing, we know that robots can be extremely fast, reliable, and precise, as for example, automated soldering robots. Hence, the idea is to replace or assist the surgeon with robotics.

Today, robotics in otologic surgery can be used for two different goals:

- Access: Reach the target structure in a minimally invasive manner.
- Assist: Execute certain surgical steps, e.g., insertion of electrodes/implants.

Both require specific technical implementations which adapt to the anatomical situation and the surgical procedure. Different benefits are promised with the use of these robotic systems and De Seta et al. [2] provide a systematic literature review that we extend in the following sections:

9.2.1 Accuracy

Accuracy and repeatability are certainly both, the most important requirements and the most important value propositions of robotics and industrial robots such as the KR CYBERTECH nano family from KUKA (KUKA Aktiengesellschaft, Augsburg, Germany) offer extremely high repeatability of 0.04 mm but they do not name any accuracy numbers publicly [3].

The achieved accuracy must match with the dimensions of the anatomical structures and the procedure. For example, the CyberKnife® system from the company Accuray Incorporated (Sunnyvale, CA, USA) for cancer treatments, using a KUKA robot, can "[achieve] accuracy of 0.5 mm manually is impossible" [4]. In order to profit from a high mechanical accuracy, the question is how to steer the robotic system toward the target and away from structures at risk. In other fields of surgery, the answer is usually to employ some image-based approach such as endoscopic vision, CT, MRI, fluoroscopy together with a master-slave robotic setup. However, in neurotologic surgeries that require drilling through or in the temporal bone with an accuracy better than 0.5 mm, endoscopic or microscopic vision does not provide the necessary foresight or might not be possible and the MRI resolution is too limited. This is one reason why master-slave systems have not had success in neurotology, though there have been attempts [5]. Therefore, the answer is usually some form of image-based planning on intraoperative CT data and a navigation setup or using a stereotactic system. This idea is feasible because the temporal bone can be used as the reference and all the structures, namely the cochlea, the nerve canals, the ossicles, etc. are in a fixed relation to the temporal bone itself. Unfortunately, the surgical navigation systems available on the market today do not deliver sufficiently high accuracy to safely navigate in the temporal bone [6]. Nonetheless, these systems can be helpful in assisting the surgeon. Consequently, custom-developed special purpose navigation systems have been suggested to overcome this limitation [7]. Labadie et al. [8] pioneered the use of a mini-stereotactic system to transfer the image-based planning to the patient coordinates, skipping cumbersome setup and registration of navigation systems. Figure 9.2 shows exemplary a CBCT scan which has been fused with a MRI scan and the level of detail that is possible to achieve today clinically.

9.2.2 Minimally Invasiveness

Another promise of robotics in neurotology is that the conventional open surgery under visual inspection can be replaced by a tiny canal in order to provide access to a target structure, e.g., the inner ear or a tumor which has been identified preoperatively. It is a fundamental principle in modern medicine to be as minimally invasive as possible in the most literal meaning of the word, which is to conserve healthy tissue as much as possible. The surgeon is limited to a working space which allows movements of instruments and provides visualization of the situs. Minimally invasive robotic/stereotactic approaches, for instance, can drill access tunnels through the mastoid with a radius of only 0.75 mm [9].

We expect that this extreme minimally invasiveness, compared to a conventional mastoidectomy, will lead to clinically relevant benefits to the patients, such as potentially shorter skin incisions, less bleeding, less risk of infection, better ability for pressure equalization due to a smaller air volume that is connected to the middle ear cavity, reduced risk of injuring the dura and other risk structures. Additionally, a dip in the skin can form above the cavity of the mastoidectomy, which can be psychologically and cosmetically relevant for the patients and it can cause issues with wearing glasses or behind-the-ear hearing aids.

Common to all minimally invasive approaches in the temporal bone is that target structures and trajectories can be identified and defined in imaging data, e.g., the

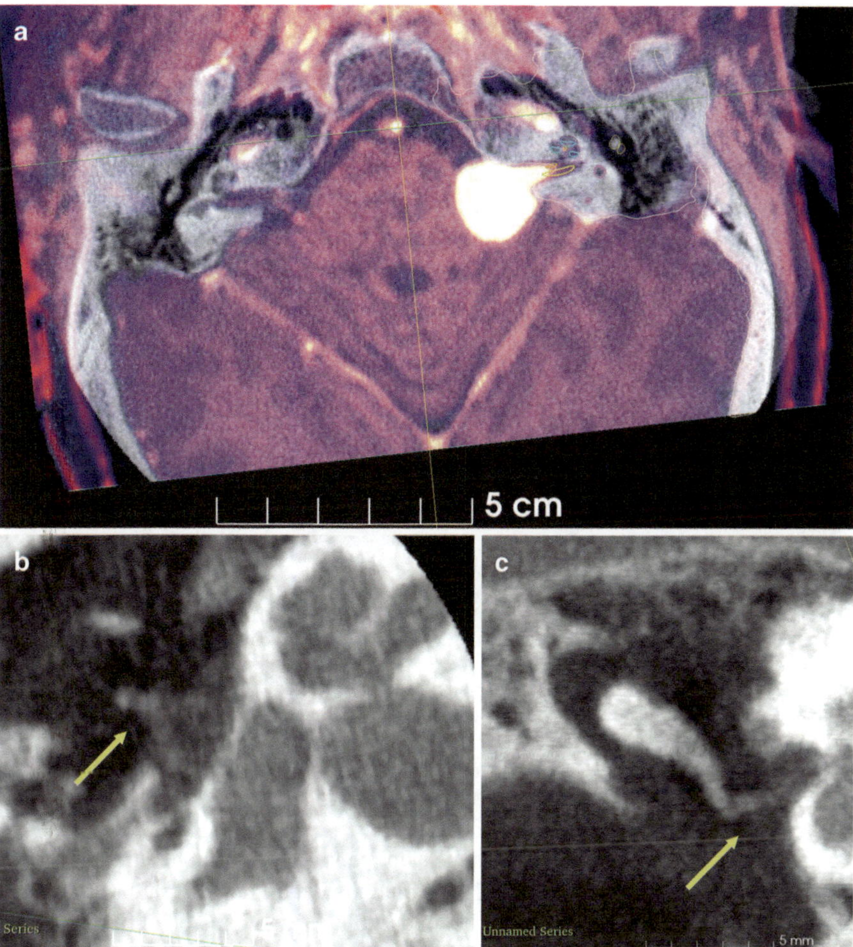

Fig. 9.2 (**a**) Modern CBCT and MRI imaging (shown here after image registration; also known as "image fusion" with false colors of the MRI scan). The CBCT scan has a 0.3-mm isometric voxel size. The MRI scan has a voxel size of 0.5 x 0.5 x 1 mm. On the right side of the image, a large tumor can be seen on the MRI scan. (**b**) A CBCT can show details in the bony structures in the middle and inner ear. A multi-planar reconstruction in the orientation of the stapes and a max-projection with a slice thickness of three voxel has been applied to display the fine structure of the stapes (yellow arrows). (**c**) The reticular process of the incus and the connection of the stapes can be identified in a 0.08-mm isometric reconstruction of a clinical CBCT device 3D Accuitomo 170 (J. MORITA CORP, Osaka, Japan)

drill path to the cochlea from the surface of the mastoid as depicted in Fig. 9.3. Improved high-resolution cone beam computed tomography (CBCT) [10, 11] can be used for this task. CBCT can provide a voxel size down to 0.1 mm, for example, with the intraoperative Xoran xCAT iQ (Xoran Technologies, Ann Arbor, USA) or even down to 0.08 mm for the 3D Accuitomo 170 (J. MORITA CORP, Osaka,

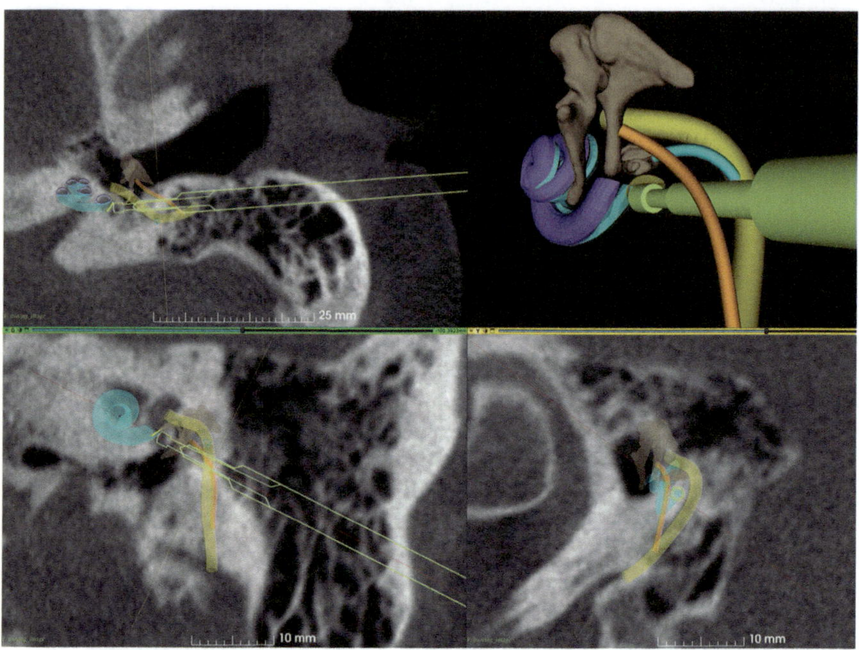

Fig. 9.3 Image-based planning for a minimally invasive surgery with the OtoJig system. First, the risk and target structures are semi-automatically segmented and 3D models are constructed and visualized in the top-right. The view can be aligned anatomically (axial, sagittal, coronal) or in line with the planned access path to be drilled or aligned along the intrinsic orientation of the cochlea. Different drill bits and their outline are overlaid in the planning

Japan). Small bony structures such as the stapes and variations in the microanatomy of the cochlear can be visualized [12]. The imaging of soft tissue structures has been also improved using MRI but is still beyond 100 µm. Image fusion allows localization of pathological processes within bony structures as shown in Fig. 9.2. Most surgical procedures require accuracy within these limits. However, some critical structures such as the basilar membrane in the inner ear cannot be visualized with the current imaging technologies. A sufficient high resolution and geometrically undistorted imaging of critical structures is a prerequisite for identification and segmentation of the relevant anatomical structures and these requirements rule out the usage of MRI for image-based planning of minimally invasive (robotic) drilling of an access tunnel to the middle or inner ear.

9.2.3 Individualization

A 3D planning of the procedure allows for virtual surgery, for example, to virtually place and shape individual implants according to the anatomic situations or to plan an intervention for precise tumor resection using different approaches (Fig. 9.3).

This preoperative information can be used intraoperatively in order to direct the robot or guide an instrument with a stereotactic system. A navigation system could be used to check every single step of the procedure at any time or it could be used to enable further assistance like augmented reality through a digital (Munich Surgical Imaging GmbH, Munich, Germany) or digital-robotic microscope (BHS Technologies GmbH, Innsbruck, Austria).

A clinically very important individualization in cochlear implantation is the individual implant placement and insertion direction according a pre-planning. A navigation system or a stereotactic system can be used to realize the patient-specific trajectory and a good alignment to the orientation of the basal turn of the cochlea is beneficial but is hard to impossible to accomplish free hand [13]. One reason for this limitation in CI is that the orientation of the cochlear is not fully visible to the surgeon but this information can be derived from pre- or intraoperative imaging.

9.2.4 Automation

Robotics will allow—at least to some degree—an independence from individual skill of the surgeon and their manual skills and thereby we believe guidance systems will deliver repeatability that can raise the quality level of the performed surgeries. A higher degree of automation with well tested and simple to use robotic or especially with stereotactic systems might lead to a better scheduling and standardization of the surgical procedure, its duration, and quality. For example, some patients exhibit a particularly dense mastoid part of the temporal bone and conventional milling requires a prolonged mastoidectomy.

9.2.5 Control

Providing guidance to access the target structure, even with a simple passive insertion tube for cochlear insertion, can limit or remove any undesired sidewards movements, drift, and tremor compared to free hand CI insertion [14]. Actuated forward movements additionally allow for a defined, constant slowness [15], potentially with force-feedback control during insertion in order to avoid trauma associated with a spike in intra-cochlear fluid pressure [16]. Notably, there is a development of a force-sensing manual insertion tool [17].

9.2.6 Better Outcomes, Potentially

It is a topic of current research how much the before mentioned properties might be able to contribute to improved outcomes, in particular, to better-hearing preservation and speech understanding in CI implantation. Outcome and complication rate in surgery are dependent on the number of procedures done by each surgeon per time. A minimum number is required to develop a routine and get experience to deal also with special cases. Robotic procedures are often pre-planned, can be double checked, and are then repeatable under constant conditions. This can reduce the intra- and inter-surgeon variability of the procedure. Barriat et al. [18] demonstrated in an experimental ex vivo setting that improved structure preservation is associated with robotic cochlear insertion. However, the clinical outcomes of a clinical group of five patients implanted with the RobOtol® robot (see below for details) compared with a group of 17 patients manually inserted, remain inconclusive in our opinion. The depth of electrode insertion was actually deeper in the manual group (416 degrees vs. 396 degrees) and the lowest hearing loss caused by the implantation was in the "no trauma" group of the manual insertion (10.86 ± 5.51 dB PTA hearing loss) compared to the "no trauma" group using the robot (13.6 ± 7.70 dB PTA hearing loss). However, in the manual insertion group, 10 patients were implanted with an abnormally bowed contour of the electrode array with an estimated elevation of the osseous spiral lamina and this group had an inferior outcome (20.50 ± 7.66 dB PTA hearing loss). Overall, we cannot yet say with certainty that a robotic electrode insertion leads to improved hearing preservation. Potentially other factors like the optimally aligned insertion trajectory, soft electrodes, the careful opening of the round window membrane, and the guidance of the electrode lead during insertion are more important to hearing preservation than just the constant slowness of the insertion forward movement alone. However, even where Heuninck et al. [19] performed robotic cochlear access with an assumingly optimally drilled trajectory, they had to conclude that "Clinical outcomes in robot-assisted cochlear implant surgery are comparable to conventional cochlear implantation."

9.2.7 Training, Education, and Remote Surgery

The use of robotics in the field of neurotology has just started. The potential for training and education has still to be elucidated and its impact on results of the surgical procedures validated through clinical studies. It is thinkable that with robotic systems, with digital and connected microscopes or endoscopes, a surgery can be accompanied or even performed by an experienced surgeon located remotely, using virtual reality.

9.3 Potential Fields of Application

The potential fields of robotic and/or stereotactic approaches are in cochlear implantation (later in this chapter), endoscopic procedures, approaches to the petrous apex, approaches to the internal auditory meatus, bone resections, stapesplasty, reconstruction of the ossicular chain, and future auditory nerve implants.

The improved diagnostics of inner ear disorders requires also perilymph sampling to identify biomarkers and underlying pathobiochemical processes. With an increasing number of available biologicals and other biological treatments, the local therapy directly of the inner ear by injecting into the perilymph becomes more and more important. In order to do both procedures, sampling and local drug delivery with high precision, e.g., volume to be administered in a range of about 1–2 μl and to avoid additional damage to the inner ear the high accuracy of the robotic system is required.

Stapesplasty is one of the most successful surgical procedures in otology. It corrects the fixed stapes in otosclerosis by replacing the natural ossicle with a stapes prosthesis. This has to be inserted very carefully into the perilymph and be securely fixed with a wire loop during the long process of the incus. In addition, the opening of the inner ear must be done with high precision, using, e.g., an otologic drill. All three steps could be done with the help of a robotic system with high accuracy avoiding less accurate manual procedures. The stapes prosthesis should be placed very slowly onto the inner ear, the fixation at the long process should be done with appropriate force to avoid losing the coupling or too strong forces on the bone of the incus which can lead to incus necrosis and subsequent recurrence of the conductive hearing loss.

In order to reconstruct the ossicular chain, mainly the incus but also a part of the malleus and the stapes have to be reconstructed using prefabricated or individually manufactured replacement prostheses. They have to be brought into position and connected with the surrounding bony structures such as the malleus handle or the stapes head or the food plate of the stapes. In order to staple prepositioning it is mandatory to conduct the necessary coupling and binding procedures using, e.g., different types of glue or cement. There will be advantages to prepositioning the prosthesis and holding it during the fixation process.

Endoscopic procedures require the reliable positioning of the endoscope within a defined anatomical region and a defined field of view. The display of this information to the surgeon and the exact positioning of the endoscope and surgical instruments cannot be done manually with the required precision. Image-guided robotic surgery could be a significant improvement in this field.

Endoscopic procedures will allow access to anatomical regions that cannot be approached through a direct path without destroying functionally important structures such as the inner ear or labyrinth. One example is the petrous apex which can be reached by a minimally invasive infralabyrinthine approach. However, the resection of the pathology requires an endoscopic procedure within a complex 3D space with important crossing or adjacent structures such as the internal carotid artery or the facial nerve.

The same is true for the internal auditory meatus. Different pathologies such as benign tumors and neurovascular compressions can be treated with a minimally invasive approach using an endoscope in addition to the microscope. The robot will allow the stable positioning of the endoscope with a given distance to the pathology and a defined angle of view.

Bone resections can be defined preoperatively as part of surgical planning. The robot can assist in precise bone removal, e.g., via a guided drill, piezoelectric instrument or a saw.

9.4 Challenges for Robotic Systems

Whether robotics can be integrated into neurotology and be widely applied depends on several factors, mainly the associated benefits and disadvantages. In the following, we list the major challenges that may hinder robotic adoption.

9.4.1 Safety

Robotic arms with multiple degrees of freedom perform drilling and implantation at the patient, and their control software must not contain malfunctions (i.e., bugs), which is a challenge given today's complexity of software projects. Also, the question of the coexistence with personnel naturally arises: Are these robots equipped with sensing capabilities to stop if a collision occurs or do all humans have to step back from the patient and interrupt their supporting activities? One proposed solution is to separate the robot from the patient by utilizing the robot for the creation of a patient-matched guiding template, and subsequently using the template to perform the surgery on the patient.

The planning of minimally invasive procedures is based on pre- or intraoperative imaging, hence the image quality and geometric correctness (free of movement artifacts, distortions, etc.) is a necessary prerequisite that has to be checked before the intervention can start. The accuracy is not only based on the imaging quality and on the mechanical properties (stiffness) of the system but also on the robustness of the navigation markers or the robustness of the bone anchoring (depending on the system design). Therefore, the image-to-patient registration should be double-checked.

9.4.2 Duration

If the set-up time to use a robotic system in the operating room or the time for the placement of (navigational) bone screws, additional imaging, planning, and registration is leading to a significant increase in the overall procedure time, the adoption of these systems will remain limited to robotic enthusiasts.

9.4.3 Complexity

The robotic system(s) should be easy to use (set up, operate, maintain) and not add to the already high mental workload of the involved personnel. Therefore, the systems should be designed to be as simple and robust as possible while also being practical to get the job done.

9.4.4 Costs

For a widespread adoption, extending beyond the leading centers, the upfront costs (invest) and the cost per surgery has to be taken into account and the additional benefit must be measured objectively and weighed against the additional costs. Expensive invests require a considerably long preparation time until funding (often public grants) can be secured and may not be in the scope of smaller hospitals. As De Seta et al. [2] wrote "There are no studies on cost analysis of the use of robotics for otological surgery. This question needs to be addressed in the future as current robots represent the most expensive devices in an ENT operating room and the cost/benefit ratio is most probably unfavorable."

9.4.5 Radiation

The most accurate and high-resolution imaging technology today is based on CT, which used ionizing radiation and correlated with the development of cancer. Thus, the use of additional scans should be minimized. However, minimally invasive drilling requires at least one scan for image-based planning and, depending on the protocol, sometimes an additional scan for an intermediate check [20]. Advancements in low-dose cone beam computed tomography (CBCT) or the development of entirely new detector technologies like single photon counting CT [21–23] will alleviate this concern and improve the precision of preoperative planning.

9.4.6 Liability

If something goes wrong, the question of who is responsible arises. Is a complication related to a malfunction of the robotic system or is it the responsibility of the surgeon entirely because they approve the planning and press (and hold) the "go" button. There will be situations where the surgeon is forced to revert to the conventional approach, and if there are complications, the question is if they were caused by the aborted robotic approach or by the following manual completion of the surgery?

9.5 Use Case: Minimally Invasive Cochlear Implantation

Cochlear implantation is nowadays a widely used treatment of choice to restore hearing in pediatric and adult patients with congenital or acquired severe to profound sensorineural hearing loss. The number of patients with serviceable residual hearing has constantly increased over the last decades and the need for hearing preservation is one of the main challenges today. Residual hearing is mainly present in the low frequencies which are represented at the apex of the cochlea while the area of the high-frequency deafness is at the basal part of the inner ear and therewith close to the round window which is the entrance path of the electrode.

Attempts to reach this goal have also uncovered the wide interindividual variability in cochlear anatomy, both in length and in shape. This has led to the concept of individualized cochlear implantation. Type, length of electrode, and insertion angle are adjusted to the anatomy and the residual low-frequency hearing of the individual patient. The desired electrode insertion depth can be precalculated. Intraoperatively, residual hearing can be monitored using cochlear monitoring with a recording of the acoustically evoked responses of the inner ear.

The current hearing preservation rate with good preservation is at about 55–70 %. Reasons for acute or delayed hearing loss are either mechanical interaction of the electrode with the micromechanics of the cochlear and/or trauma to intracochlear structures with subsequent biological trauma reaction.

However, fundamental problems of an atraumatic electrode insertion are not solved so far. The insertion of the electrode is done through either the round window or a cochleostomy but the surgeon cannot follow the electrode propagation within the cochlea. The insertion beyond the entry point into the cochlea is without visual control and does not follow the optimum trajectory to minimize intracochlear trauma.

The speed of manual insertion cannot practically be reduced below approx. 1 mm/s and is on average at 1.6 mm/s [24] which leads to insertion forces along the insertion path. Reduction of speed down to 0.1 mm/s would significantly reduce the insertion forces and avoid sudden strokes [25].

Current cochlear implantation still requires extended mastoid surgery (Fig. 9.4). Robot-assisted surgery would allow a minimal invasive surgery using a single preplanned drilled pathway from the surface of the mastoid down to the cochlea. The drilled canal will represent also the optimized trajectory for atraumatic electrode insertion. The insertion could be done through the canal using a motorized insertion system. Several implementations of this approach are already available, underdevelopment, or in clinical use.

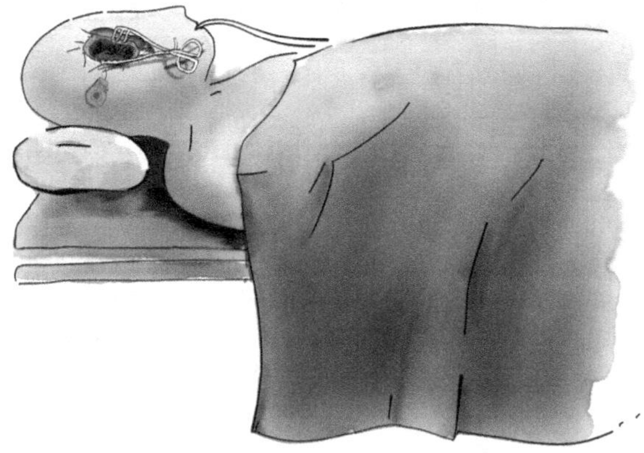

Fig. 9.4 Schematic drawing of the conventional open mastoidectomy approach for cochlear implantation. The ear is folded forward and after a skin incision, the mastoid bone is removed (mastoidectomy) in an area about 3 × 4 cm

The required accuracy is high and at the limits of today's technology, especially imaging resolution. The drill path shall keep safe distances from certain structures in order to avoid accidental damage to the facial nerve, the chorda tympani, the ossicular chain, or the wall of the external ear canal etc..

9.6 Current Implementations of Robotics in Neurotology

There is a number of robotic systems specifically designed for use in neurotology, more specifically in otology. General purpose master-slave robots do not play a role, but it has been attempted to use a Da Vinci system [5], seemingly without a clear clinical benefit, neither in minimally invasiveness nor in surgery duration.

The specific robotic systems in neurotology so far aim to support mainly cochlear implantation due to the importance of CI and due to the difficulties associated with this challenging microsurgery. These systems can be divided into two main categories:

- Devices addressing a slow, continuous, and controlled insertion speed of the cochlear implant electrode into the inner ear. However, these devices are not necessarily addressing the optimal trajectory, nor the insertion vector which would require an additional image-based planning software and navigation.
- Devices addressing the creation of safe, minimally invasive access paths through the temporal bone toward the middle or inner ear, including an option to choose or optimize the trajectory and insertion angle.

We are listing devices that are either certified medical devices or are already used in a clinical investigation, with the exception of the CochlearHydroDrive.

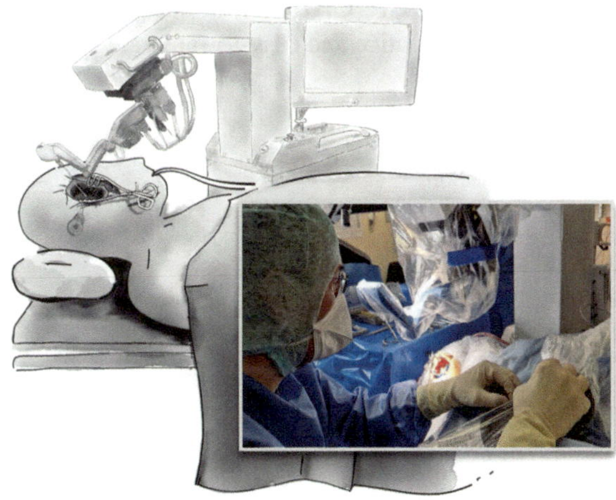

Fig. 9.5 Schematic drawing of the robotic ENT system RobOtol® of the company Collin using a CI electrode array holder to position and advance the array into the cochlea. A conventional, open surgery is necessary before the robot can be used for this application because the system needs some space to rotate around its pivot point. The system can also be used to manipulate through the external ear canal

9.6.1 Ad 1—Devices Addressing Electrode Insertion

RobOtol® Sterker and his team [26] researched and developed a robotic system with the company Collin to be used for positioning and inserting a CI electrode into the cochlea (Fig. 9.5) and potentially other applications such as stapedectomy, ossiculoplasty, and where a robotic instrument holder can be helpful. The technical concept is basically a master-slave system such that the operator steers the robotic arm around a pivot point with a space navigator (like a joystick with additional degrees of freedom). The system has 7 degrees of freedom (3 rotations, 3 translations, one distal movement) and can produce slow and constant movement speeds. RobOtol is advertised as a platform to support more types of applications and is commercially available as a medical device according to the medical device directive (MDD, Council Directive 93/42/EEC of 14 June 1993). Coupled with a navigation system, the system could even be used to attempt a suitable insertion axis for cochlear implantation as described by Torres et al. [27].

iotaSOFT™ Insertion System Iotamotion is a commercial company offering a small single-use FDA-approved device to be sold for conventional open cochlear implantation with the goal to insert a cochlea implant electrode array via round window or via cochleostomy approach into a radiographically normal cochlea and allowing to control the speed of electrode insertion. The device shall be fixated, during the surgery, at the skull surface (Fig. 9.6). The hypothesis is that a steady, constant, slow insertion speed of 0.1 mm/a leads to 51 % lower insertion forces with 78 % variation compared to manual insertions of surgeons with multiple experience levels [28, 29]. If and to what degree the expected lower insertion forces and variations might translate to objectively measurable hearing preservation is a much anticipated future publication.

CochlearHydroDrive(CHD) From our group [30, 31], there is a research prototype for a cost-effective and easy-to-integrate system that is using an infusion pump

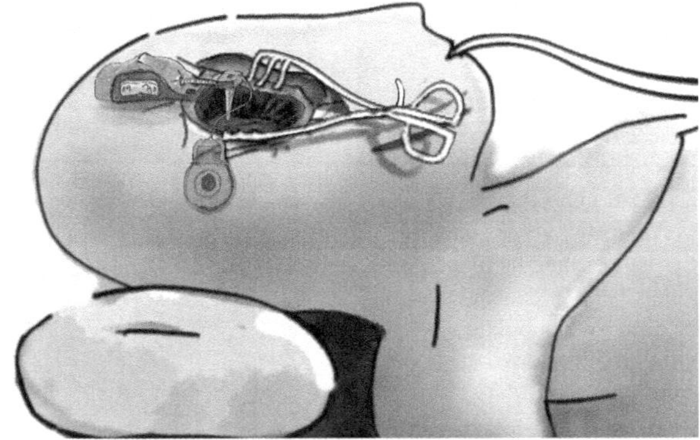

Fig. 9.6 Schematic drawing of the disposable (single-use) iotaSoft actuator, transiently screwed to the patient's skull, for holding and advancing CI electrode arrays at extremely slow speeds. A conventional, open surgery is necessary before the system can be used as intended. The device is compatible with multiple CI electrodes

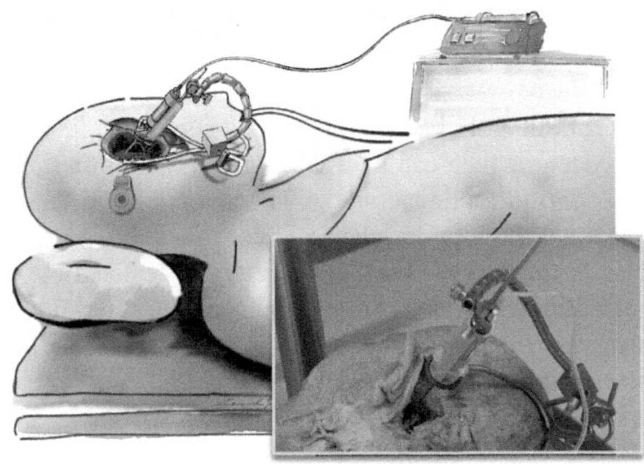

Fig. 9.7 Schematic drawing of our research prototype, using an infusion pump and a syringe to produce a constant and slow forward movement and push a CI electrode array forward into the cochlea

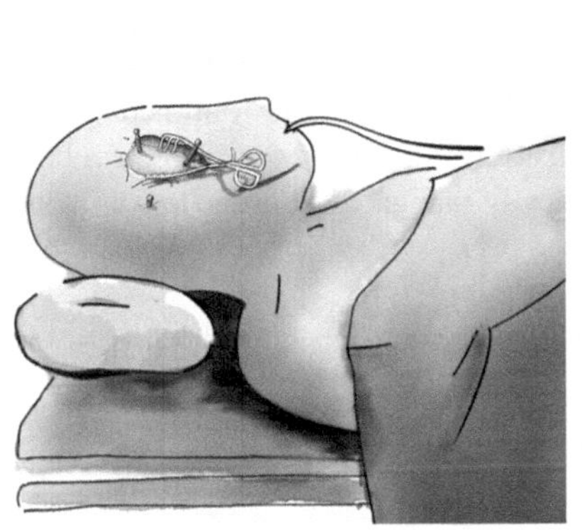

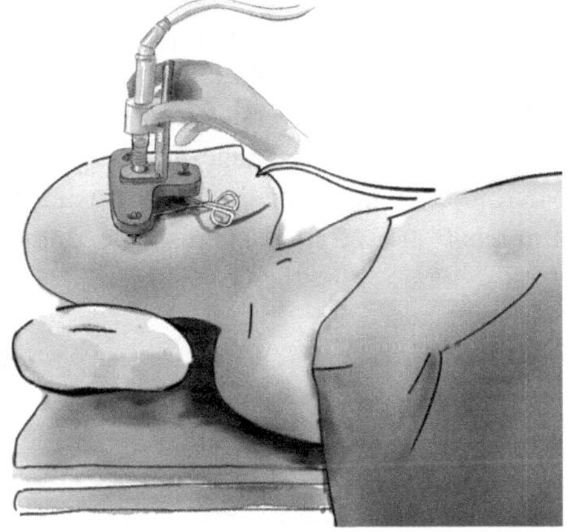

Fig. 9.8 Schematic drawing of the Microtable® microstereotactic frame and drill press for drilling minimally invasive access tunnels to the cochlea. Left: In the first step, there are three bone-anchored extenders with spherical sphere markers. These can be identified in a computed tomography scan in order to perform image-based planning of the trajectory. Right: On a milling machine, a t-shaped template is customized such that three through-holes are created that fit to the positions of the three fiducial markers. Each hole has a different depth step inside which is used to define the angle of the template. After sterilization, the customized template is attached with three grippers to be put into the drilled holes. The grippers connect to the fiducial markers. In an additional central through hole, a drill press can be inserted to guide a surgical drill for the minimally invasive access

to produce an extremely slow forward movement for automated electrode insertions (Fig. 9.7). As Rau et al. wrote "a first prototype of a tool with maximum simplicity was designed and fabricated to take advantage of hydraulic actuation. The prototype facilitates automated forward motion using a syringe connected to an infusion pump." This device claims to produce speeds as low as 0.03 mm/s.

9.6.2 Ad 2—Devices Addressing Creating a Minimally Invasive Access to the Inner Ear

Microtable® Labadie et al. [32] pioneered the idea of a bone-anchored stereotactic system, which can be used to guide the drilling of an access tunnel toward the inner ear, in a clinical study. The authors write "A customized microstereotactic frame was rapidly designed and constructed to constrain a surgical drill along the desired trajectory" and this trajectory is realized by pre- and intraoperative computed tomography (CT) to use the bone-anchored fiducial markers for image-based planning (Fig. 9.8). Since Labadie et al. reported a facial nerve paresis caused by heat during drilling, the research such as Feldmann et al. [33] has moved away from the usage of high-speed surgical drills.

Hearo CAScination is developing a robotic system marketed as "Hearo" based on earlier research by Bell et al. [7]. The feasibility of the application for robotic middle ear access in patients that have a facial recess of at least 2.5 mm in width has been reported by Caversaccio et al. [20]. The basic idea is to use bone screws as fiducial markers for image-guided planning similar to the one outlined for the Microtable®, however, instead of using a customized drilling template, a robotic arm has to be set up, draped sterile, and optically navigated in order to follow the

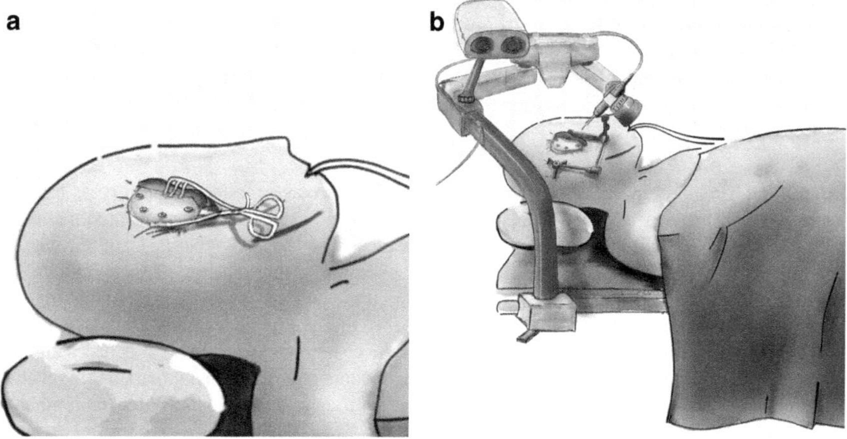

Fig. 9.9 Schematic drawing of the Hearo setup. (**a**) There are four bone screws to be placed behind the pinna. These will be identified as fiducial markers in an intraoperative cone beam computed tomography CBCT scan for image-guided planning. (**b**) Additional to the bone screws, there is a clamping device with an optical marker screwed to the skull, so that a stereo-camera can be used as a navigation system. The robotic arm needs to be mounted onto the rails of the patient bed and registered to the patient coordinates by steering the robotic arm to touch the four screw heads one after another. Once this setup procedure has been completed and given the optical marker has not moved, the robot can perform a safe minimally invasive drilling according to the pre-planned trajectory

planned trajectory (Fig. 9.9). Please refer to chapter "Robotics for Approaches to the Mastoid/Mastoidectomy" for further details on the numerous steps to prepare, set up, and conduct a Hearo-procedure.

ROSA® robotic system (Amiens, France) is an attempt to adapt an already available 6 degree-of-freedom robot used for neurosurgical applications to perform minimally invasive cochlear implantation including electrode array insertion. A pilot clinical study reported principle feasibility when a safety margin of 2.5 mm is kept [34].

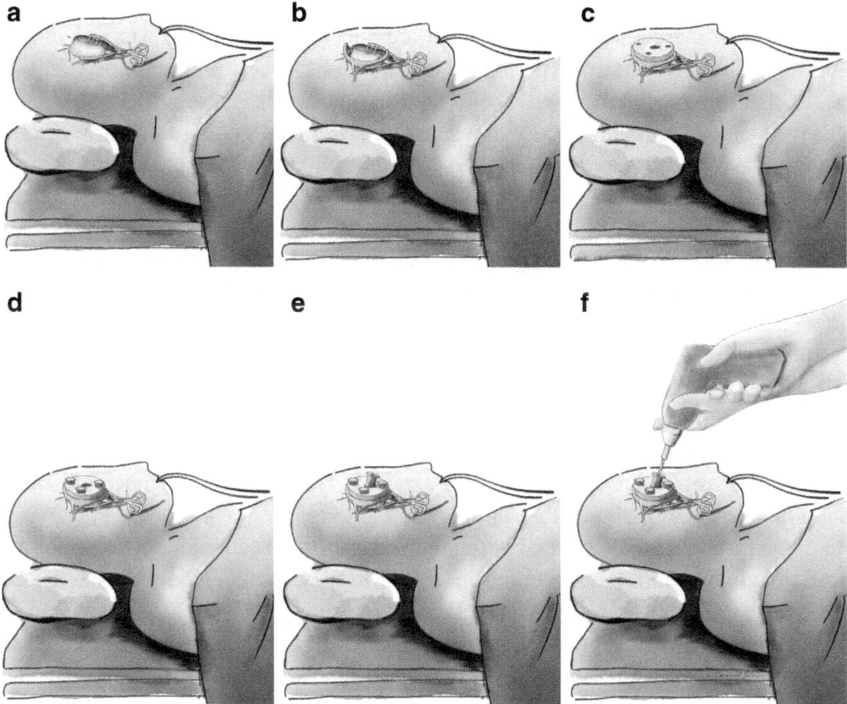

Fig. 9.10 Schematic drawing of the OtoJig procedure. (**a**) Preparation of the situs and skin incision. (**b**) A reusable frame is attached with a single bone screw and a computed tomography scan is performed for image base planning. (**c**) A patient-matched single-use positioning jig is produced near the operating theater on an automated manufacturing machine. The position, angle, and depth of a through-hole define the individually planned trajectory relative to the frame. (**d**) Jig fasteners are clicked into the jig for fixation. (**e**) A tool guide is inserted into the through-hole (this can also be done in step c). (**f**) A spiral drill bit is intended to be used with a battery-powered drill unit to create the minimally invasive inner ear access

OtoJig Our group at MHH researched an improved mini-stereotactic concept that is based on patient-matched positioning jigs to guide the minimally invasive drilling. The whole system is designed for safety and simplicity [9]. As a safety-by-design, the "robot" in this system is not acting at the patient's head but is an automated manufacturing machine comprising of a hexapod robot and a drill unit that customizes the disposable positioning jigs according to the planning. The positioning jig receives a through a hole in the defined position and angle according to the image-based planning [35]. For the surgical procedure at the patient, a single bone screw is required for the fixation of the mini-stereotactic frame, which is used for registration purposes and as well for the guiding drill bits and tools (Fig. 9.10).

9.7 Future Developments

Robots or robotic systems will gradually play a role in neurotology and as clinical evidence might potentially show improved outcomes in the foreseeable future, the adoption will increase even though there are concerns regarding costs and surgery duration. The most innovative opinion leaders and forward thinking hospitals will be the first to pave the way and create scientific/medical evidence.

For cochlear implant surgery, the separately realized goals of creating a minimally invasive access and a controlled insertion will converge and in this area we will likely see adoption of task-specific robotic and precision surgery. More systems are coming to market in this area. With intraoperatively available imaging systems such as impedance spectroscopy or fluoroscopy in order to guide and position electrodes into the inner ear, the "blindness" of using a key-hole procedure will be alleviated. Partly, the steps for bone-fixating registration markers, CT imaging, and planning could eventually be performed under local anesthesia such that the duration of intervention that needs to be performed in the operating theater might be completed within 15 minutes of time. This would allow a very efficient outpatient treatment due to the expected shorter downtime and recovery of patients.

A similar robotic progress might be expected for crimping of stapes prosthesis and to control the force and the supply onto the loop.

In the future, we believe, that with the availability of even higher resolution low-dose imaging technologies, robotics in neurotology will enable individualized minimally invasive precision surgeries far beyond the capabilities of the human hand for normal anatomy and some—but not all—challenging cases. However, a universal autonomous neurotologic robotic system does not seem feasible and the most successful systems will aim to assist instead of replace the surgeon.

Declaration of Conflict of Interest TL and SJ declare being limited partners of HörSys IP GmbH & Co. KG which holds a financial stake in OtoJig GmbH, which is a German company that owns and further develops the described technology, SJ is the CEO of OtoJig.

References

1. Andersen, B., Bandel, P., Bartlog, J., Feiler, A., Gisch, S., Janß, A., Kasparick, M., Keller, A., Matzke, G., Rosenau, L., Schlichting, S. (2020). Medical device approval based on the SDC participant key purpose standards for safe interoperability. https://ornet.org/wp-content/uploads/2020/10/PKP-technical-report-v1.1.pdf.
2. De Seta D, Daoudi H, Torres R, Ferrary E, Sterkers O, Nguyen Y. Robotics, automation, active electrode arrays, and new devices for cochlear implantation: a contemporary review. Hear Res. 2021:108425. https://doi.org/10.1016/j.heares.2021.108425.
3. KUKA, KR CYBERTECH nano. 2023. https://www.kuka.com/en-us/products/robotics-systems/industrial-robots/kr-cybertech-nano. Accessed 14 Feb 2023.
4. Muacevic, A.. Virtual knife: precise treatment of tumors and metastases with robots. KUKA website. 2020. https://www.kuka.com/en-us/industries/solutions-database/2020/02/cyberknife. Accessed 14 Feb 2023.
5. Liu WP, Azizian M, Sorger J, Taylor RH, Reilly BK, Cleary K, Preciado D. Cadaveric feasibility study of da Vinci Si-assisted cochlear implant with augmented visual navigation for otologic surgery. JAMA Otolaryngol Head Neck surg. 2014;140(3):208–14. https://doi.org/10.1001/jamaoto.2013.6443.
6. Majdani O, Rau TS, Baron S, et al. A robot-guided minimally invasive approach for cochlear implant surgery: preliminary results of a temporal bone study. Int J CARS. 2009;4:475–86. https://doi.org/10.1007/s11548-009-0360-8.
7. Bell B, Stieger C, Gerber N, Arnold A, Nauer C, Hamacher V, et al. A self-developed and constructed robot for minimally invasive cochlear implantation. Acta Otolaryngol. 2012;132(4):355–60.
8. Labadie RF, Mitchell J, Balachandran R, Fitzpatrick JM. Customized, rapid-production microstereotactic table for surgical targeting: description of concept and in vitro validation. Int J Comput Assist Radiol Surg. 2009;4:273–80.
9. Salcher R, John S, Stieghorst J, Kluge M, Repp F, Fröhlich M, Lenarz T. Minimally invasive Cochlear implantation: first-in-man of patient-specific positioning jigs. Front Neurol. 2022;13:829478. https://doi.org/10.3389/fneur.2022.829478.
10. Leung R, Chaung K, Kelly JL, Chandra RK. Advancements in computed tomography management of chronic rhinosinusitis. Am J Rhinol Allergy. 2011;25(5):299–302.
11. Scarfe WC. Cone beam computed tomography: volume acquisition. White and Pharoah's Oral Radiology E-Book: Principles and Interpretation: Second South Asia Edition E-Book, 150; 2019
12. Pietsch M, Schurzig D, Salcher R, et al. Variations in microanatomy of the human modiolus require individualized cochlear implantation. Sci Rep. 2022;12:5047. https://doi.org/10.1038/s41598-022-08731-x.
13. Torres R, Kazmitcheff G, Bernardeschi D, De Seta D, Bensimon JL, Ferrary E, Nguyen Y. Variability of the mental representation of the cochlear anatomy during cochlear implantation. Eur Arch Otorhinolaryngol. 2016;273:2009–18.
14. Riojas KE, Labadie RF. Robotic Ear surg. Otolaryngol Clin N Am. 2020;53(6):1065–75.
15. Rajan GP, Kontorini G, Kuthubutheen J. The effects of insertion speed on inner ear function during cochlear implantation: a comparison study. Audiol Neurootol. 2013;18(1):17–22.
16. Banakis Hartl RM, Greene NT. Measurement and Mitigation of Intracochlear Pressure Transients During Cochlear Implant Electrode Insertion. Otol Neurotol. 2022 Feb 1;43(2):174-182. https://doi.org/10.1097/MAO.0000000000003401. PMID: 34753876; PMCID: PMC10260290.
17. Böttcher-Rebmann G, Schell V, Budde L, Zuniga MG, Baier C, Lenarz T, Rau TS. A tool to enable intraoperative insertion force measurements for Cochlear implant surgery. IEEE Trans Biomed Eng. 2022;70:1643. https://doi.org/10.1109/TBME.2022.3224528.
18. Barriat S, Peigneux N, Duran U, Camby S, Lefebvre PP. The use of a robot to insert an electrode array of cochlear implants in the cochlea: a feasibility study and preliminary results. Audiol Neurotol. 2021;26(5):361–7. https://doi.org/10.1159/000513509.

19. Heuninck E, Van de Heyning P, Van Rompaey V, et al. Audiological outcomes of robot-assisted cochlear implant surgery. Eur Arch Otorhinolaryngol. 2023; https://doi.org/10.1007/s00405-023-07961-7.
20. Caversaccio M, Wimmer W, Anso J, Mantokoudis G, Gerber N, Rathgeb C, Scheider D, Hermann J, Wagner F, Scheidegger O, Huth M, Anschuetz L, Kompis M, Williamson T, Bell B, Gavaghan K, Weber S. Robotic middle ear access for cochlear implantation: first in man. PLoS One. 2019;14(8):e0220543. https://doi.org/10.1371/journal.pone.0220543.
21. Hsieh SS, Leng S, Rajendran K, Tao S, Mc Collough CH. Photon counting CT: clinical applications and future developments. IEEE Trans Radiat Plasma Med Sci. 2021;5(4):441–52. https://doi.org/10.1109/trpms.2020.3020212. Epub 2020 Aug 28. PMID: 34485784; PMCID: PMC8409241
22. Taguchi K, Iwanczyk JS. Vision 20/20: single photon counting x-ray detectors in medical imaging. Med Phys. 2013;40(10):100901. https://doi.org/10.1118/1.4820371.
23. Iwanczyk JS, Nygard E, Meirav O, Arenson J, Barber WC, Hartsough NE, et al. Photon counting energy dispersive detector arrays for x-ray imaging. IEEE Trans Nucl Sci. 2009;56(3):535–42.
24. Kontorinis G, Lenarz T, Stöver T, Paasche G. Impact of insertion speed of cochlear implant electrodes on the insertion forces. Otol Neurotol. 2011;32:565–70.
25. Todt I, Mittmann P, Ernst A. Intracochlear fluid pressure changes related to the insertional speed of a CI electrode. Biomed Res Int. 2014;2014:507241.
26. Miroir M, Nguyen Y, Szewczyk J, Mazalaigue S, Ferrary E, Sterkers O, Bozorg Grayeli A. RobOtol: from design to evaluation of a robot for middle ear surgery. In: Proceedings of the IEEE/RSJ International Conference on Intelligent Robots and Systems, vol. 2010; 2010. p. 850–6.
27. Torres R, Kazmitcheff G, De Seta D, Ferrary E, Sterkers O, Nguyen Y. Improvement of the insertion axis for cochlear implantation with a robot-based system. Eur Arch Otorhinolaryngol. 2017;274(2):715–21.
28. iotamotion. Company website, front-page. 2023. https://iotamotion.com/. Accessed 1 Feb 2023
29. Kaufmann CR, Henslee AM, Claussen A, Hansen MR. Evaluation of insertion forces and cochlea trauma following robotics-assisted Cochlear implant electrode Array insertion. Otol Neurotol. 2020;41(5):631–8.
30. Rau TS, Zuniga MG, Salcher R, Lenarz T. A simple tool to automate the insertion process in cochlear implant surgery. Int J Comput Assist Radiol Surg. 2020;15(11):1931–9.
31. Geraldine Zuniga M, Lenarz T, Rau TS. Hydraulic insertions of cochlear implant electrode arrays into the human cadaver cochlea: preliminary findings. Eur Arch Otorhinolaryngol. 2022;279(6):2827–35. https://doi.org/10.1007/s00405-021-06979-z.
32. Labadie RF, Balachandran R, Noble JH, Blachon GS, Mitchell JE, Reda FA, Dawant BM, Fitzpatrick JM. Minimally invasive image-guided cochlear implantation surgery: first report of clinical implementation. Laryngoscope. 2014;124(8):1915–22.
33. Feldmann A, Anso J, Bell B, et al. Temperature prediction model for bone drilling based on density distribution and in vivo experiments for minimally invasive robotic Cochlear implantation. Ann Biomed Eng. 2016;44:1576–86. https://doi.org/10.1007/s10439-015-1450-0.
34. Klopp-Dutote N, Lefranc M, Strunski V, Page C. Minimally invasive fully ROBOT-assisted cochlear implantation in humans: preliminary results in five consecutive patients. Clinical otolaryngology: official journal of ENT-UK; official journal of Netherlands Society for Oto-rhino-laryngology & Cervico-facial. Surgery. 2021;46:1326. https://doi.org/10.1111/coa.13840.
35. Rau TS, John S, Kluge M, Repp F, Geraldine Zuniga M, Stieghorst J, Timm ME, Fröhlich M, Majdani O, Lenarz T. Ex vivo evaluation of a minimally invasive approach for Cochlear implant surgery. IEEE Trans Biomed Eng. 2023;70(1):390–8. https://doi.org/10.1109/TBME.2022.3192144.

The Future of Robotics in Skull Base Surgery

10

Abigail Reid, Daniel Prevedello, Douglas Hardesty, Ricardo Carrau, and Kyle Van Koevering

10.1 Introduction

Although robotics are typically associated with STEM fields today, the word robot actually originated from a play written by Karel Capek, which was first performed in 1921 [1]. The Czech word *robota* translates to slave labor, and the play, *Rossum's Universal Robots*, told the story of robot servants performing tedious tasks for humans and the revolution that followed [2]. Despite early descriptions of robots in the arts, it was not until decades later that robots became scientifically realized [1] with the invention of the Unimate, the first industrial robot. After at, industrial use of robots grew exponentially, and almost 25 years after the invention of Unimate the PUMA 560 (Westinghouse Electric Corporation, Pittsburgh, PA, USA) became the first surgical robot to be used in 1985 [1].

While definitions of robots vary, primarily because of disagreements regarding whether robots require artificial intelligence and autonomous function, three main types of robotic systems have been identified within the field of surgery [2]. Active systems work autonomously to complete pre-programmed tasks. Semi-autonomous systems use pre-programmed tasks in conjunction with surgeon control. Master-slave systems such as the da Vinci Surgical System (Intuitive Surgical, Sunnyvale, CA, USA) are operated entirely by the surgeon and are characterized by a complete lack of autonomous function.

A. Reid
Creighton University School of Medicine, Omaha, NE, USA

D. Prevedello · D. Hardesty
Department of Neurosurgery, Ohio State University, Columbus, OH, USA

R. Carrau . K. Van Koevering (✉)
Department of Otolaryngology-Head and Neck Surgery, Division of Skull Base Surgery and Division of Head and Neck Oncology, Ohio State University, Columbus, OH, USA
e-mail: Kyle.vankoevering@osumc.edu

M. M. Al-Salihi et al. (eds.), *Robotics in Skull-Base Surgery*, https://doi.org/10.1007/978-3-031-38376-2_10

Since the invention of the PUMA 560, major advances have been made in the field of surgical robotics including the landmark development of the da Vinci system. Today, their use has become standard in urological, gynecological, and general surgery [3]. Surgical robotics have been optimized for these fields allowing their use in many procedures to become standard practice. Unfortunately, the bony constraints of the skull base present challenging limitations not seen in the abdomen or pelvis and have made the use of currently available robotic surgical systems difficult in these anatomical regions.

Current research on skull base robotic surgery has mainly used the da Vinci surgical system to compare surgical approaches to the skull base in cadavers and rare clinical studies. While one of the goals of surgical robotics is to allow for minimally invasive procedures, current tools are large in comparison to the preferred entry points to the skull base such as the nostril. As a result, while cadaver models can prove feasibility, they often fail to provide a purely minimally invasive method of approaching the skull base. While research is performed with currently available technology, new robotic surgical systems are in development and offer hope based on features that include the incorporation of haptic feedback and decreased robotic arm size [4, 5].

In addition to the development of novel surgical robotics, research is being conducted on various applications including telesurgery, image guidance systems, and the automation of surgical robots using machine learning models [6]. While much research will be needed prior to clinical adoption of these applications, the many advantages they could provide offer an exciting glimpse into the future of skull base robotic surgery and the field of robotic surgery as a whole.

10.2 Current State of Surgical Robotics

One of the first robotic surgical systems to be used and arguably the most popular to date is the da Vinci Surgical System. The introduction of the da Vinci, which features 3D visualization, tremor filtration, and wrist-like movements, marked the beginning of a massive push for adoption of robotic systems in many surgical fields [2]. While tremor filtration increases the degree of precision, 3D visualization and increased degrees of freedom potentially mimic the advantages of open surgical techniques. The degrees of freedom provided by the EndoWrist technology used in the da Vinci system are particularly advantageous because they provide greater maneuverability than conventional endoscopic instruments [7]. While conventional endoscopic instruments provide insertion, rotation, pitch, yaw, and grip for a total of five degrees of freedom, the da Vinci has external arms that provide insertion, pitch, and yaw in addition to the EndoWrists that provide internal pitch, yaw, rotation, and grip, for a total of seven degrees of freedom (Fig. 10.1). However, despite the many potential advantages of surgical robotics, their widespread use has been limited to only a few disciplines: urology, gynecology, and general surgery, with more recent applications in neurosurgery and otolaryngology. That said, the proposed future

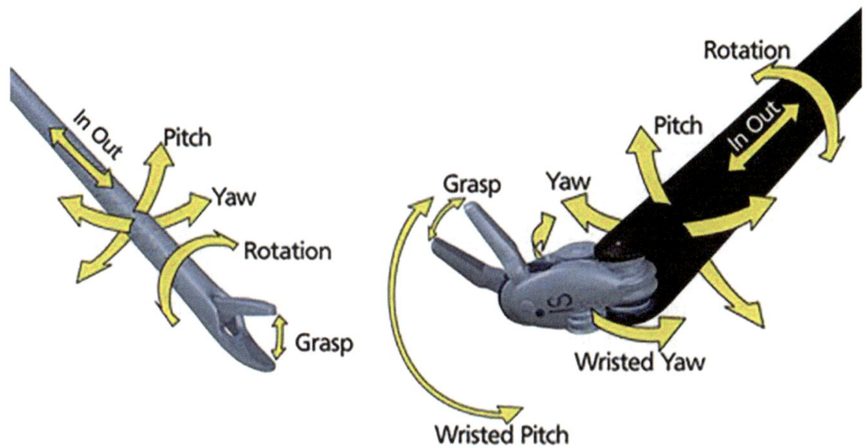

Fig. 10.1 Comparison of movement capabilities in endoscopic and robotic instrumentation. Conventional endoscopic instruments (left) provide five degrees of freedom while the da Vinci EndoWrist (right) allows for seven degrees of freedom due to the hinged wrist at the working end of the instrument

applications of surgical robotics extend far beyond this list of specialties. Notably, while the EndoWrist has not been approved by the FDA for use in the skull base, the increase in degrees of freedom available will probably be an important design requirement for the development of skull base-specific robotic equipment.

10.2.1 Applications of Robotic Surgery in Urological, Gynecological, and General Surgery

Urological, gynecological, and general surgery are currently leaders in the clinical application of robotic surgery. In 2000, the first robot-assisted prostatectomy was performed, followed by formal FDA approval for the procedure 1 year later [8]. Previously, most prostatectomies were performed as open procedures; since then, robotic-assisted prostatectomies have increased dramatically. In fact, robotic-assisted radical prostatectomy increased from 13.6% to 72.6% between 2003 and 2012 [9]. In addition to radical prostatectomy, urological robot-assisted procedures include radical cystectomy and partial nephrectomy [10]. Following a few years behind urological applications of robot-assisted surgical devices, the FDA approved the use of the da Vinci in gynecological surgeries in 2000 [11]. Since then, the da Vinci has become a standard tool in several gynecological procedures such as hysterectomy, myomectomy, oophorectomy, endometriosis treatment, sacrocolpopexy, and tubal anastomosis. Lastly, there is a growing use of surgical robots in general surgery including inguinal and ventral hernia repair and cholecystectomies [12].

10.2.2 Applications of Robotic Surgery in Neurosurgery and Otolaryngology

While a few fields have embraced surgical robotics, skull base neurosurgery and otolaryngology have been slower to adopt these new technologies despite the precision that surgical robots could lend to the field in technically difficult and repetitive tasks [13]. Currently, robotics in neurosurgery are primarily used in conjunction with imaging to provide navigation assistance, a technique that has grown in popularity owing to the fragility of structures in the brain and spine. Clinical applications include intracranial biopsy, pedicle screw placement in spinal surgeries, and placement of intracranial leads such as in stereoelectroencephalography and deep brain stimulation. Presently, only two surgical systems are under active use and development in cranial neurosurgery [14]. Neuroarm (IMRIS, Deerfield, MN, USA) uses intraoperative magnetic resonance imaging to provide image guidance during procedures. 3D images of the surgical site, haptic feedback, and the ability of the robotic arms to use microsurgical tools are additional features of the system. One potential drawback is the requirement for intraoperative MRI capabilities, which are absent in many operating rooms. The ROSA System (Zimmer Biomet, Warsaw, IN, USA) also uses image guidance and haptic feedback and has been shown to improve accuracy while minimizing risks. This system allows for pre-operative planning using MRI data and can perform tasks autonomously with surgeon oversight or be directly controlled. In 2021, a study was published on the use of Laser Interstitial Thermal Therapy (LITT) ablation of a posterior fossa mass using a customized 3D implant that highlighted the benefit of a tool such as ROSA for pre-operative planning of LITT procedures on difficult-to-reach masses [15]. One of the largest studies on the use of robotic support in pediatric neurosurgical cases was published in 2017 [16]. In this study, 128 procedures were performed using the ROSA system including electrode implantation for stereoelectroencephalography, stereotactic biopsy, neuroendoscopy, pallidotomy, shunt placement, deep brain stimulation, and stereotactic cyst aspiration. The study outcomes supported the use of the ROSA system owing to its safety and the minimization of postoperative morbidity, with a surgical success rate of 97.7% in the 128 procedures studied and an early clinical transient complication rate of 3.9%. This indicates that the use of ROSA in neurosurgery will probably continue to grow in the coming years.

While neurosurgery has been somewhat slow to adopt robotic systems, otolaryngology, and specifically head and neck, has seen a more rapid increase in the use of robotics since the FDA approved application of the da Vinci for transoral robotic surgery (TORS) in 2009 [5]. Since then, TORS has been investigated for use in several head and neck applications, specifically oropharyngeal, hypopharyngeal, and laryngeal disease through the minimally invasive transoral approach. In fact, TORS has become a widely accepted method for treating oropharyngeal squamous cell carcinoma (SCC) and presents several advantages over alternative treatment options. While TORS has found most success in the treatment of oropharyngeal SCC, application of this method is also under investigation for treating obstructive sleep apnea, thyroid and parathyroid diseases, laryngeal lesions, and sublingual and submandibular gland diseases, and for diagnosing carcinomas with unknown primaries [5, 17].

10.3 Current Research on Skull Base Robotic Surgery

While robotic surgery is becoming the standard of care in some specialties because of its enhanced precision and ability to perform procedures with minimally invasive access, skull base surgery has notably lagged. Major obstacles to adoption involve the complex anatomy of the skull base combined with the narrow anatomical corridors of typical access points relative to currently available surgical robotic systems [18]. Current research on robotics in skull base surgery most commonly uses the da Vinci system and investigations primarily involve approaches to the skull base in cadaver and limited human studies to explore the advantages, limitations, and areas of need in skull base robotic surgery.

10.3.1 Advantages and Limitations of Robotics in Skull Base Surgery

While the limitations of currently available technology have restricted the clinical feasibility of skull base robotic surgery, robotics in this setting has many potential advantages. As the most popular system, the da Vinci will serve as the main robotic system for analyzing the advantages and limitations of robotics in skull base surgery.

The da Vinci system provides 3D visualization, seven degrees of freedom, and tremor filtration in addition to enhancing surgical ergonomics [18, 19]. Altogether, robotics in surgery provides the potential for minimally invasive procedures that could improve patient health and cosmetic outcomes. The increased precision provided by the excellent visualization, maneuverability, and tremor filtration of surgical robotics has the potential to increase the safety of such procedures and could obviate the need for many commonly performed open procedures in the future.

While the potential advantages of robotic skull base surgery are exciting and promising, numerous limitations will need to be addressed in next generation surgical robotics before they can be realized clinically. Additionally, a cost-benefit analysis will be needed to determine whether the cost of the surgical robotics, training, and maintenance is outweighed by enhanced patient outcomes and safety.

As previously stated, the da Vinci system was not originally created for application in the skull base. As a result, several major limitations will need to be addressed in future iterations of novel surgical robotic systems before minimally invasive robotic skull base surgery can be adopted clinically. Systematic reviews of the current state of research in robotic skull base surgery have revealed a number of these key limitations [18–20]. Perhaps most problematic is the size of the da Vinci arms, which are markedly larger than those used in standard endoscopic endonasal procedures. While standard endoscopes are 4 mm in diameter, EndoWrist instrumentation is currently available in 5 mm and 8 mm sizes [21, 22]. This difference has made it incredibly challenging to find a suitable approach to the skull base that remains minimally invasive. Another limitation is the lack of a drill in currently available da Vinci systems. Drills are frequently used in skull base operations, and without incorporation of such a tool these procedures require all drilling to be performed bedside by a second surgeon. A third limitation is the lack of haptic feedback in the da Vinci system. While the visualization provided by surgical robotics is excellent, work on the skull base with its complex and delicate structures would benefit significantly from tactile feedback, which is not currently available. Until such feedback is readily incorporated, delicate work around critical neurovascular structures is likely to be deemed unsafe by most skull base surgeons.

10.3.2 Robotic Approaches to the Skull Base

Currently, skull base robotics is limited by access through the nostrils with available instrumentation. As such, accessory ports have been described, primarily through cadaveric dissection. The feasibility of robotic-assisted endoscopic surgery of the skull base was first studied in 2007 using a transantral approach on four cadavers to access the central and anterior skull base in order to ensure proper closure of dural defects [23]. Since then, several studies have been published exploring novel approaches to the skull base in an attempt to realize the many potential advantages of robotic surgery that have been largely limited in this anatomical region to date. Below we will review some of the primary approaches to skull base robotics by access technique.

10.3.2.1 Transnasal Approach

Most research on robotics in skull base surgery has used the da Vinci system with alternative approaches to the skull base. Although the da Vinci is widely available, with several design advantages, the diameter of the arms along with restrictions on maneuverability within the relatively small nasal cavity make it unsuitable for a pure transnasal approach to the skull base [20]. Therefore, although a transnasal approach to the skull base is theoretically appealing, very little research has been done on this approach using robotics. One proposed solution is to use the Flex System (Medrobotics, Raynham, MA, USA) [24], which enables compatible flexible instruments of only 3.5 mm diameter to be used and provides visualization using an endoscope with an HD camera system and 180 degrees of flexibility. Notably, the Flex System also provides haptic feedback to the surgeon, which is currently unavailable in the da Vinci system.

While the study of pure transnasal access successfully explored the potential for the Flex System in skull base pathology, the method involved partial removal of the septum and midfacial degloving on four cadavers (Fig. 10.2), so it is not ideal for

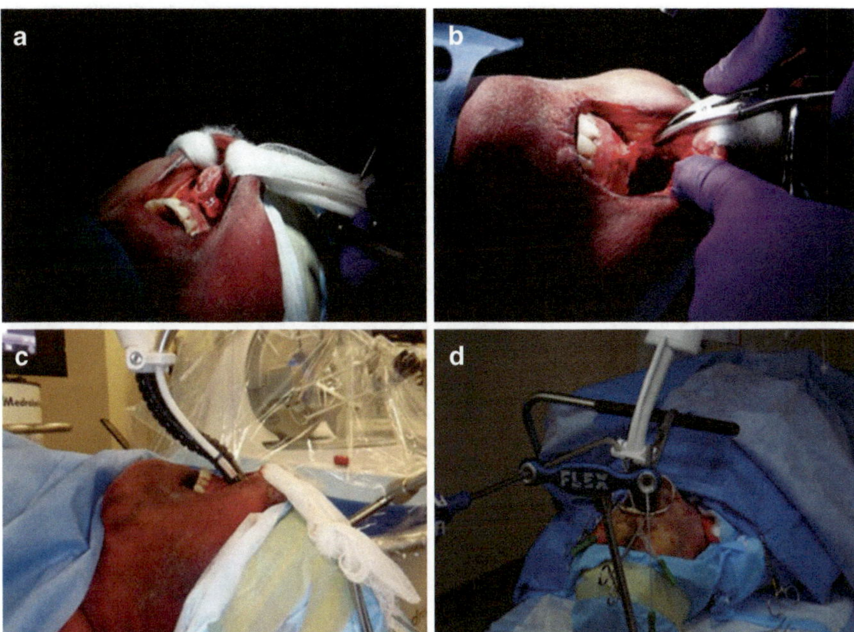

Fig. 10.2 Flex Robot access through midface degloving approach. Although a transnasal route would theoretically provide the ideal access to the skull base, current systems are too bulky to work within the confines of the nostrils. Additional access options include a modified midfacial degloving and b resection of parts of the maxillary frontal recess and nasal septum with bilateral medial turbinectomy. After surgical preparation for transnasal access, c endoscopic endonasal visualization is employed followed by d introduction of compatible flexible instruments to the skull base

clinical use [24]. Future research will be needed to create less invasive procedures using the Flex System for a pure transnasal approach to be feasible.

10.3.2.2 Transoral Approach

Among the currently researched approaches, transoral is among the most prevalent [19]. The aperture being much wider than the nose, a combined transoral approach can accommodate larger instruments while maintaining the desired minimally invasive techniques with no incisions additional to alternative approaches. Early transoral approaches used transpalatal incisions to increase visualization in several cadaver and human studies [25–27]. However, with decreases in the size of the da Vinci arms, a transoral approach without palatal incisions has also become feasible [20] (Fig. 10.3). In fact, in 2016, Chauvet et al. became the first group to report on the clinical use of a purely transoral robotic approach for removing sellar tumors in four patients [28]. However, a major limitation of the transoral approach is that access is largely limited to the nasopharynx, sphenoid, and sella.

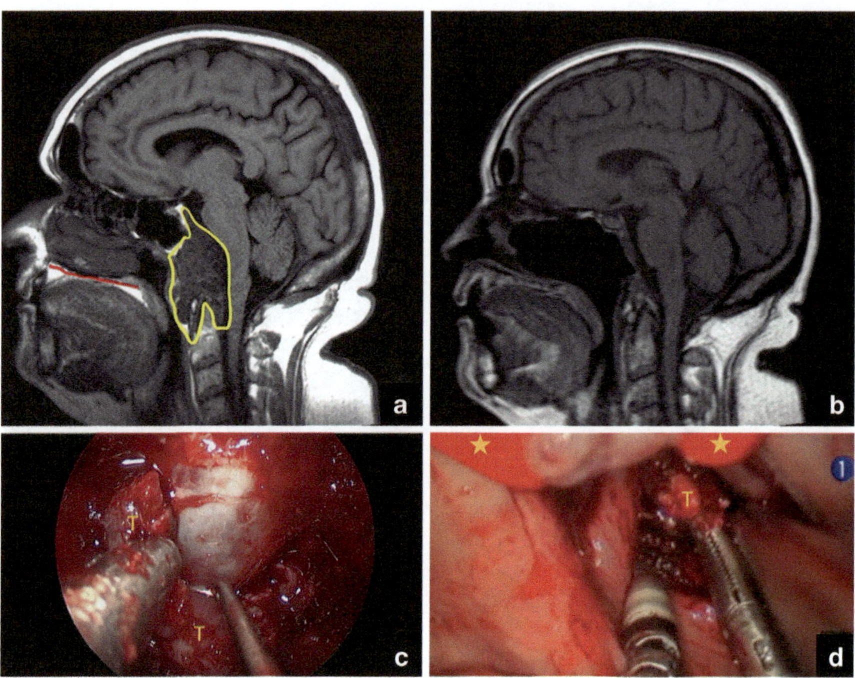

Fig. 10.3 Transoral Robotic-assisted Nasopharyngectomy for clival chordoma. (**a**) The chordoma (outlined in yellow) involves the entirety of the clivus and into C1 and the retropharyngeal space. The hard palate (outlined in red) creates a bony limit to inferior extension with conventional endoscopic instruments. (**b**) MRI after removal of the chordoma via a transoral approach. (**c**) Endoscopic Endonasal Approach allowed for the tumor to be peeled from the pre-pontine dura, but could not access the most inferior portion of the tumor. (**d**) Transoral Assistance with the da Vinci enabled the remaining tumor to be removed because of articulating instrumentation (T = Tumor; * = red rubber catheter retracting the soft palate)

10.3.2.3 Supraorbital and Transorbital Approaches

The supraorbital keyhole approach is a minimally invasive technique for accessing the skull base. While the small incisions are beneficial for patients, they limit instrument movement and visualization for the surgeon, including the added difficulty of working around the supraorbital nerve. Robot surgical systems have been proposed as a way to mitigate these limitations [29, 30]. While greater dexterity has been achieved for the supraorbital keyhole approach using the da Vinci surgical system, conflicting opinions regarding safety and feasibility remain. One large limitation remains the narrow access point that prohibits the simultaneous use of endoscope and instruments. This makes it likely that adoption of this method will require novel surgical robotics better suited to the narrow access points used in skull base operations.

An alternative solution has been investigated in a study that involved both transorbital and transnasal access to the skull base [31]. This approach was used to avoid some of the space limitations encountered in singular methods of approach and resulted in an increased range of angles between instruments. This study was performed using computer simulation, dry skulls, and cadaver models; further investigations will be required to determine the clinical feasibility and safety of this approach.

10.3.2.4 Transantral Approach

A few studies have also been performed using cadaver models to prove the feasibility of transantral approaches to the skull base using the da Vinci. A major potential advantage of robotics in the skull base is the potential for suture closure of dural defects through minimally invasive surgeries [32]. In 2011, Kupferman et al. used a bilateral transmaxillary approach to repair dural defects successfully in four fresh frozen cadaveric heads using robotic-assisted techniques. This approach enabled the anterior skull base to be reconstructed. Two years later, Blanco and Boahene studied approaches to both the anterior skull base and the infratemporal area [33]. The anterior skull base was accessed using transmaxillary and nasal corridor approaches in combination. While the approach was successful, researchers noted that the size of the da Vinci arms placed limitations on maneuverability even after surgical expansion of the nasal corridor. Altogether, while a transantral approach to the skull base is feasible, redesigned surgical robotics will be necessary to optimize the approach and will include distal articulating tips and miniaturization of the robot arms to enhance use in skull base regions.

10.3.2.5 Transcervical Approach

Transcervical approaches have been tested with some success in combination with transoral or transnasal cameras [34]. They provide an excellent range of motion and instrument maneuverability. In the transcervical approach, trocars are inserted close to the angle of the mandible though a paramandibular incision, while the optic lens is inserted either transorally or transnasally. Unfortunately, the lack of a drilling tool in the da Vinci system remains a major hindrance to this and other techniques to access the skull base. Dallan et al. have also investigated transcervical approaches to the skull base [35]. In this study, combined transcervical-transnasal access was achieved and was determined to be superior to transcervical-transoral approaches for dissection of the posterior skull base in cadaveric models on the basis of enhanced visualization. Despite increases in range of motion and maneuverability, no clinical cases have been reported to date.

10.4 Envisioning the Future of Robotic Surgery

The potential advantages of robotic surgery have made adoption of new technology in operating rooms promising for surgeons, patients, and innovators. As some of Intuitive Surgical's (Sunnyvale, CA, USA) restrictive patents have begun to expire and new technologies become available, we are likely to see a shift in the surgical robotic system market. Already, many new systems are being developed and are preparing to undergo the process of FDA approval. Additionally, new technology in other sectors including augmented reality and artificial intelligence has begun to be incorporated into surgical systems. While technologies such as telesurgery and programmed robotic surgeries were once considered science fiction, current research suggests that these applications of robotics will become feasible in the foreseeable future.

10.4.1 Novel Surgical Robotic Systems

Currently available surgical robotics have revolutionized surgery over the past two decades. That said, remaining areas of need include incorporation of haptic feedback and drilling instrumentation, reduction in cost and surgical arm size, increased flexibility, and further studies proving the benefits of surgical robotics in relation to their cost. Up to this point, the da Vinci surgical system has championed the surgical robotic market. However, over the last decade or so, novel robotic systems have been in development across the world and are potential competitors in the market. Several of these newer surgical robotics will be described in what follows, chosen primarily on the basis of their potential for direct use in skull base surgery or for specific desired features in these surgeries (Table 10.1).

10.4.1.1 Flex Robotic System

The Flex Robotic System is currently used in head and neck surgery and was approved by the FDA in 2015 after being developed specifically for use in TORS procedures [5]. Unlike some robotic systems, the Flex system was designed as a

Table 10.1 Comparison of surgical robotic systems with regard to application in the skull base

Robotic system	Advantage	Disadvantage
da Vinci	Seven degrees of freedom, 3D visualization, tremor filtration	Cost, lack of haptic feedback, relatively large instrumentation, lack of drill
Flex	Haptic feedback, rigid and flexible camera state options, lower cost, smaller instrumentation, compatible flexible instrumentation, increased access	Requires 3D goggles, optics less sharp than da Vinci, hybrid system uses manually controlled instrumentation rather than robotics
Senhance	Eye tracking, haptic feedback, reusable easily moved instruments	Bulky equipment, lack of articulating instruments
Versius	Five-wristed robotic arms, haptic feedback, lower cost	No FDA approval, limited current applications
REVO-I	Comparable design to the da Vinci at lower cost	No FDA approval, limited current applications, less experience
SPORT	Multi-articulated instruments, single port design increases accessibility	Currently in research and development phase
Concentric tube robot	Design optimized to size constraints and bony anatomy increasing MIS accessibility, size, flexibility, and maneuverability ideal for skull base	Currently in research and development phase

hybrid system with a flexible robotic endoscope and manually controlled instrumentation. Some of its advantages over the da Vinci include incorporation of haptic feedback, the option of either rigid or flexible states, increased access thanks to smaller instrumentation, and lower cost. Although originally designed for use in head and neck surgery, the device has since been used in general surgery and gynecology, further proving the benefit attainable from more flexible robotic designs that address the access and line of sight problems that limit many current robotic systems [36]. While the Flex system requires 3D goggles and provides worse optics than the da Vinci, the haptic feedback is a notable advantage for head and neck surgeries [36]. Moreover, the Flex system provides easier access to cancers of the larynx, distal tongue base, and hypopharynx that were previously difficult or impossible to resect using TORS, and it has been shown to be both safe and reliable.

10.4.1.2 Senhance Surgical Robotic System

Two years after the approval of Flex, the Senhance Surgical Robotic System (Asensus Surgical, Durham, NC, USA) received FDA approval in 2017 [4]. While bulky equipment size and lack of articulating instruments mark pain points for this system, the incorporation of eye tracking to control the camera system based on eye focus and head movements make it particularly intriguing. Additional features include incorporation of haptic feedback, seven degrees of freedom in each of three arms mounted on individual carts, and reusable instruments with easy replacement thanks to a magnetic attachment design. Currently, the Senhance system is used primarily in gynecological and colorectal procedures, but applications could expand as research on this system continues [5].

10.4.1.3 Versius Robotic System

The Versius Robotic System (CMR Surgical, Cambridge, United Kingdom), which is currently used in Europe for colorectal, gynecological, renal, and upper GI surgeries, is awaiting FDA approval in the USA [4, 5]. This modular system uses up to five different wristed robotic arms with the incorporation of haptic feedback and compatibility with 5 mm instruments. It is estimated to be more cost-effective than currently commercially available systems, offering hope for continued cost reduction in surgical robotics in the future.

10.4.1.4 REVO-I Surgical Robotic System

In 2015, the South Korean Meere Company introduced the REVO-I surgical robotic system (Meere Company, Hwaseong, Gyeonggi-do Province, South Korea) [37]. This system is similar to the da Vinci and could be a future competitor in the American market pending FDA approval given the similar capabilities combined with reduced cost of the REVO-I system [38]. The REVO-I system is far newer the da Vinci so its applications are currently limited. In Korea, REVO-I has been used primarily for cholecystectomy and a few cases of appendectomy. That said, given the similarities between the two systems, the REVO-I is likely to follow a similar trajectory of expanding surgical applications to the da Vinci as more research is performed.

10.4.1.5 Single Port Orifice Robotic Technology Surgical System

The Single Port Orifice Robotic Technology (SPORT) (Titan Medical, Chapel Hill, NC, USA) is a surgical system currently under development and boasting access-related advantages similar to systems such as the da Vinci SP and the Flex Robotic System, both of which are single port systems [4, 5]. While not yet FDA approved, SPORT has reported success in animal models. The SPORT design consists of a single port 25 mm in size through which two multi-articulated instruments can be inserted.

10.4.1.6 Concentric Tube Robot System

One robotic system of particular interest here is a concentric tube robot that originated in the MED Lab at Vanderbilt University. This device involves curved telescoping tubes that can bend and elongate, featuring movements of needle-sized arms that are described as tentacle-like [39]. This system was built specifically for transnasal robotic skull base surgery so its design is optimized for the size constraints and intricacy of the anatomy involved. In 2015, this technology was used in a phantom study of endonasal skull base tumor removal [40]. Several years later, it was used in a phantom study for transnasal removal of orbital tumors [41]. Both studies proved successful and offer an exciting glimpse into future applications of concentric tube robots in surgery. While designed for transnasal usage for skull base tumors, this technology has the potential for use in many different areas of the body that are currently difficult or impossible to reach with commercially available surgical robotics.

10.4.2 Image Guidance and Augmented Reality

Image guidance and the application of augmented reality in surgery have become topics of study and debate over the past decade as technological capabilities improve, but the lack of cost-benefit analyses makes further development and adoption challenging. Notably, a number of studies have been published investigating the value of image guidance and augmented reality in head and neck surgical cases including TORS and cochlear implantation [42–46]. One current limitation of image guidance and augmented reality involves registration, a step that effectively marks areas of the patient (typically using bony landmarks or surface anatomy) so the computer can track them and display instrumentation and 3D overlays properly. Unfortunately, intraoperative shift of tissue is not uncommon and can result in inaccuracies in image guidance and augmented reality applications [47]. To address this problem, research is being performed to develop a deformable registration algorithm using cone beam computed tomography (CBCT) [45]. This research was performed in TORS of the tongue base and showed the feasibility of the technique and the advantages of augmentation, which included relevant vasculature and desired resection data. While further study of registration accuracy will be required, this marks an important step toward implementing image guidance and augmented reality technology in head and neck procedures. Another relevant study showed the feasibility of incorporating augmented reality into cochlear implantation procedures using the da Vinci in a cadaveric model [44]. Although much research will be required to develop and ensure its accuracy and safety, this technology has the potential to improve patient outcomes and change medical education in surgery.

10.4.3 Telesurgery

The origin of the da Vinci system and surgical robotics as we know them today actually stemmed from the desire to implement remote surgical procedures on military personnel and astronauts [2]. Accordingly, early versions of this technology received heavy funding from NASA. Telesurgery involves the remote control of master-slave robotic systems. In principle, these surgeries could be performed from extremely remote locations provided the set-up is established appropriately on site. This was tested for the first time in 2001 by a team in New York, USA on a patient in Strasbourg, France [48]. Unfortunately, several limitations including latency time, lack of haptic feedback, cost, cybersecurity threats, equipment acquisition, and legal/billing issues and public skepticism have severely restricted the clinical application of telesurgery since then [48, 49]. That said, several potential advantages of telesurgery are worth considering. These include the elimination of long-distance travel, providing healthcare to medically underserved populations, encouraging surgical collaborations, and addressing surgeon shortages [49]. With advances in network speeds, development of haptic feedback in surgical robots, and new robotics entering the market, potentially reducing cost, there is hope that we can take advantage of these benefits more fully in the coming decades, ensuring a future in which safe, minimally invasive, surgical care is trusted and widely available. That said, the push for robotic automation could make telesurgery irrelevant in the future as active robotic systems are improved and commercialized, potentially reducing the need for long distance control of master-slave systems.

10.4.4 Surgical Robotic Automation

The development and application of machine learning models and automation have increased enormously over the past 10 years. However, while autonomous robots grow in popularity and use, the feasibility of implementing them in surgery remains uncertain. Industrial automation requires the creation of robots that perform repetitive, predictable tasks. Such robots do not require the incorporation of machine learning models. In contrast, surgical robotics will require the ability to sense and respond to novel situations appropriately, thereby requiring the development of machine learning models for these applications. This ambitious goal will require careful consideration of surgical skills and the methods that can be used to analyze them, improved understanding of the safety and reliability of autonomous systems, and a thorough understanding of how robots adapt to new challenges [50]. Beyond the technical issues presented by the development of autonomous surgical robotics, researchers, and innovators should be prepared to address problems and thus gain acceptance and trust from the public as well as physicians. Despite the many current limitations and areas of research, machine learning offers exciting opportunities for the future of surgical robotics.

Currently, a few robotic surgical systems are programmable or aid in surgical decision-making including CyberKnife (Accuray, Sunnyvale, CA, USA), Mako SmartRobotics (Stryker, Kalamazoo, MI, USA), and Yomi (Neocis, Miami, FL, USA) [51]. CyberKnife uses real-time imaging during treatment to concentrate radiation at the site of the lesion while reducing the extent of injury to healthy tissue and adjusting for slight movements throughout the procedure [52]. Mako SmartRobotics is currently used for total knee, total hip, and partial knee replacements [53]. It involves precision surgical planning based on patient scans that reduce resection of healthy tissue and provides a data analytics component for comparing outcomes and identifying areas of improvement. Lastly, Yomi is used in dentistry for procedure planning and uses augmented anatomical visualization and haptic feedback [54]. These are just a few surgical robotics that have begun the process of incorporating real-time patient-specific data into decision-making and serve as the basis for surgical robotic innovation and automation in the future. While current technology offers more limited results than the promises of fully autonomous systems, these systems serve as proof of concept for the feasibility and benefits that can be achieved in the future. Ultimately, the goal of machine learning models in surgical robotics is to train the robots to perform a vast library of surgical skills competently, thus enabling the robot to complete surgical procedures from start to finish with minimal or no intervention from surgeons. While initial surgical robotics will be developed as semi-autonomous and involve skills and eventually procedures that are repetitive and fairly predictable, robots will eventually gain both autonomy and complexity through the use of machine learning [50].

10.5 The Idealized Skull Base Robotic Surgery

Robotic surgery has undergone remarkable advances over the past two decades since the FDA approval of the da Vinci in 2001. Although there is currently no ideal surgical robotic system for use in the skull base, increased adoption of robotic surgical systems, increased development of novel systems, and further development of current systems promise a bright future for skull base robotic surgery. While the development of such a system will take time, many of the key features are already in research and development stages. The first and most obvious feature required for adoption of skull base robotic surgical procedures will be enhanced and miniaturized instrumentation. The Concentric Tube Robot System [39] is one example of a technology that could be applied to an ideal system given its potential for addressing problems of small access points and bony constraints and allowing for a purely transnasal approach. Another feature of an ideal system will include the seven degrees of freedom for instruments, which provides much of the benefit of current robotic systems. Tremor filtration and 3D visualization are also important features to maintain with additional instrumentation including drills, Doppler, and nerve stimulators. Seamless integration with operative navigation will allow radiographic reference to the instrument's location to be made at all times. Haptic feedback will be another crucial feature given the delicate bony drilling performed in skull base surgery and will serve to increase the safety and precision of these procedures. Another feature that could increase safety and precision is the use of augmented reality to create digital 3D overlays of key neurovascular structures to assist with surgeon identification. Other ideal features would include telesurgery capabilities and eventually robotic automation, facilitating access to these surgical techniques for which there is inadequate training in different areas of the world or a potential shortage of surgeons. Lastly, the cost of an ideal system such as the one described, and of robotic surgical systems more generally, could benefit from significant reduction. Currently, there are major concerns regarding the cost of acquisition, maintenance, and training regarding the da Vinci and other surgical robotic systems [55]. While further analysis of the costs and benefits of robotic surgery compared to traditional approaches could mitigate some of these concerns, overall reduction in the cost of these systems will enable their use to be more easily justified and ultimately allow for clinical realization of their many potential benefits.

10.6 Conclusion

Currently, clinical use of robotics in skull base surgery is incredibly limited. However, with exciting new developments in surgical robotics and related technology, the potential benefits and applications cannot be overstated. While the da Vinci is currently the leading robotic surgical system, major limitations including size and lack of haptic feedback have not allowed for clinical adoption in many specialties. Through research into several approaches to the skull base using the da Vinci and other surgical robotic systems, these limitations have been thoroughly explored and clearly require either advances over the current design or novel robotic systems built specifically for the skull base. Since several of Intuitive Surgical's patents are expiring and research has shown the need for advances in robotics, we are likely to continue to see the development and approval of surgical robotic systems. Judging from the current technology and rapidly evolving research interests, it is likely we will see the integration of robotics into skull base surgery in the near future. Some advances that will make this possible include incorporation of haptic feedback, miniaturization of instruments, and flexible instrument and scope options that will increase access. In addition to addressing the limitations identified, future advances are likely to include applications such as telesurgery, image guidance, and surgical robotic automation. Although ambitious, these advances will enable skull base surgeries to be performed in a minimally invasive manner, potentially ensuring shorter recovery time, better outcomes, and enhanced precision while also preparing for a future in which robots can perform surgeries remotely and autonomously for safe, widely available care.

References

1. Badaan SR, Stoianovici D. Robotic systems: past, present, and future. In: Hemal AK, Menon M, editors. Robotics in genitourinary surgery. London: Springer; 2011. p. 655–65. https://doi.org/10.1007/978-1-84882-114-9_59.
2. Lane T. A short history of robotic surgery. The Annals of The Royal College of Surgeons of England. 2018;100(6_sup):5–7. https://doi.org/10.1308/rcsann.supp1.5.
3. Leung T, Vyas D. Robotic surgery: applications. American Journal of Robotic Surgery. 2014;1(1):1–64.
4. Peters BS, Armijo PR, Krause C, Choudhury SA, Oleynikov D. Review of emerging surgical robotic technology. Surg Endosc. 2018;32(4):1636–55. https://doi.org/10.1007/s00464-018-6079-2.
5. Tamaki A, Rocco JW, Ozer E. The future of robotic surgery in otolaryngology – head and neck surgery. Oral Oncol. 2020;101:104510. https://doi.org/10.1016/j.oraloncology.2019.104510.
6. Tarassoli SP. Artificial intelligence, regenerative surgery, robotics? What is realistic for the future of surgery? Annals of Medicine and Surgery. 2019;41:53–5. https://doi.org/10.1016/j.amsu.2019.04.001.
7. Chen CCG, Falcone T. Robotic Gynecologic surgery: past, present, and future. Clin Obstet Gynecol. 2009;52(3):335–43. https://doi.org/10.1097/GRF.0b013e3181b08adf.
8. Shah J, Vyas A, Vyas D. The history of robotics in surgical specialties. American Journal of Robotic Surgery. 2014;1(1):12–20. https://doi.org/10.1166/ajrs.2014.1006.
9. Hu JC, O'Malley P, Chughtai B, Isaacs A, Mao J, Wright JD, Hershman D, Sedrakyan A. Comparative effectiveness of cancer control and survival after robot-assisted versus open radical prostatectomy. J Urol. 2017; https://doi.org/10.1016/j.juro.2016.09.115.
10. Jeong W, Kumar R, Menon M. Past, present and future of urological robotic surgery. Investigative and Clinical Urology. 2016;57(2):75–83. https://doi.org/10.4111/icu.2016.57.2.75.
11. Sinha R, Sanjay M, Rupa B, Kumari S. Robotic surgery in gynecology. Journal of Minimal Access Surgery. 2015;11(1):50–9. https://doi.org/10.4103/0972-9941.147690.
12. Intuitive | Surgeons | Robotic Assisted General Surgeons. (n.d.). Retrieved June 1, 2022, from https://www.intuitive.com/en-us/healthcare-professionals/surgeons/general
13. Khanna O, Beasley R, Franco D, DiMaio S. The path to surgical robotics in neurosurgery. Operative Neurosurgery. 2021;20(6):514–20. https://doi.org/10.1093/ons/opab065.
14. Elsabeh R, Singh S, Shasho J, Saltzman Y, Abrahams JM. Cranial neurosurgical robotics. Br J Neurosurg. 2021;35(5):532–40. https://doi.org/10.1080/02688697.2021.1950622.
15. Kozlowski J, VanKoevering K, Heth JA. A customized 3D implant to target laser interstitial thermal therapy ablation of a posterior fossa mass. J Clin Neurosci. 2021;90:238–43. https://doi.org/10.1016/j.jocn.2021.05.064.
16. Benedictis AD, Trezza A, Carai A, Genovese E, Procaccini E, Messina R, Randi F, Cossu S, Esposito G, Palma P, Amante P, Rizzi M, Marras CE. Robot-assisted procedures in pediatric neurosurgery. Neurosurg Focus. 2017;42(5):E7. https://doi.org/10.3171/2017.2.FOCUS16579.
17. Cammaroto G, Stringa LM, Zhang H, Capaccio P, Galletti F, Galletti B, Meccariello G, Iannella G, Pelucchi S, Baghat A, Vicini C. Alternative applications of trans-Oral robotic surgery (TORS): a systematic review. J Clin Med. 2020;9(1):E201. https://doi.org/10.3390/jcm9010201.
18. Little AS, Mooney MA, Abel TJ, Albuquerque FC, Almefty KK, Almefty RO, Anand VK, Arnaout O, Baranoski JF, Barkhoudarian G, Benet A, Bergsneider M, Blue R, Brammli-Greenberg S, Brigeman S, Bristol RE, Carr SB, Carrau RL, Cetas JS, et al. Controversies in Skull Base surgery. Thieme Verlag. 2019; https://doi.org/10.1055/b-006-164734.
19. Pangal DJ, Cote DJ, Ruzevick J, Yarovinsky B, Kugener G, Wrobel B, Ference EH, Swanson M, Hung AJ, Donoho DA, Giannotta S, Zada G. Robotic and robot-assisted skull base neurosurgery: systematic review of current applications and future directions. Neurosurg Focus. 2022;52(1):E15. https://doi.org/10.3171/2021.10.FOCUS21505.

20. Heuermann M, Michael AP, Crosby DL. Robotic Skull Base surgery. Otolaryngol Clin N Am. 2020;53(6):1077–89. https://doi.org/10.1016/j.otc.2020.07.015.
21. Ballouhey Q, Clermidi P, Cros J, Grosos C, Rosa-Arsène C, Bahans C, Caire F, Longis B, Compagnon R, Fourcade L. Comparison of 8 and 5 mm robotic instruments in small cavities. Surg Endosc. 2018;32(2):1027–34. https://doi.org/10.1007/s00464-017-5781-9.
22. Solari D, Villa A, De Angelis M, Esposito F, Cavallo LM, Cappabianca P. Anatomy and surgery of the endoscopic endonasal approach to the Skull Base. Translational Medicine @ UniSa. 2012;2:36–46.
23. Hanna EY, Holsinger C, DeMonte F, Kupferman M. Robotic endoscopic surgery of the Skull Base: a novel surgical approach. Arch Otolaryngol Head Neck Surg. 2007;133(12):1209–14. https://doi.org/10.1001/archotol.133.12.1209.
24. Schuler PJ, Scheithauer M, Rotter N, Veit J, Duvvuri U, Hoffmann TK. A single-port operator-controlled flexible endoscope system for endoscopic skull base surgery. HNO. 2015;63(3):189–94. https://doi.org/10.1007/s00106-014-2950-1.
25. Fernandez-Nogueras FJJ, Katati MJ, Arraez Sanchez MA, Molina Martinez M, Sanchez Carrion M. Transoral robotic surgery of the central skull base: preclinical investigations. Eur Arch Otorhinolaryngol. 2014;271(6):1759–63. https://doi.org/10.1007/s00405-013-2717-4.
26. Kim GG, Zanation AM. Transoral robotic surgery to resect skull base tumors via transpalatal and lateral pharyngeal approaches. Laryngoscope. 2012;122(7):1575–8. https://doi.org/10.1002/lary.23354.
27. Ozer E, Waltonen J. Transoral robotic Nasopharyngectomy: a novel approach for nasopharyngeal lesions. Laryngoscope. 2008;118(9):1613–6. https://doi.org/10.1097/MLG.0b013e3181792490.
28. Chauvet D, Hans S, Missistrano A, Rebours C, Bakkouri WE, Lot G. Transoral robotic surgery for sellar tumors: first clinical study. J Neurosurg. 2016;127(4):941–8. https://doi.org/10.3171/2016.9.JNS161638.
29. Hong W-C, Tsai J-C, Chang SD, Sorger JM. Robotic Skull Base surgery via supraorbital keyhole approach: a cadaveric study. Neurosurgery. 2013;72:A33. https://doi.org/10.1227/NEU.0b013e318270d9de.
30. Marcus HJ, Hughes-Hallett A, Cundy TP, Yang G-Z, Darzi A, Nandi D. da Vinci robot-assisted keyhole neurosurgery: a cadaver study on feasibility and safety. Neurosurg Rev. 2015;38(2):367–71. https://doi.org/10.1007/s10143-014-0602-2.
31. Bly RA, Su D, Lendvay TS, Friedman D, Hannaford B, Ferreira M, Moe KS. Multiportal robotic access to the anterior cranial fossa: a surgical and engineering feasibility study. Otolaryngol Head Neck Surg. 2013;149(6):940–6. https://doi.org/10.1177/0194599813509587.
32. Kupferman ME, DeMonte F, Levine N, Hanna E. Feasibility of a robotic surgical approach to reconstruct the Skull Base. Skull Base. 2011;21(2):79–82. https://doi.org/10.1055/s-0030-1261258.
33. Blanco RGF, Boahene K. Robotic-assisted Skull Base surgery: preclinical study. Journal of Laparoendoscopic & Advanced Surgical Techniques. 2013;23(9):776–82. https://doi.org/10.1089/lap.2012.0573.
34. Ozer E, Durmus K, Carrau RL, de Lara D, Ditzel Filho LFS, Prevedello DM, Otto BA, Old MO. Applications of transoral, transcervical, transnasal, and transpalatal corridors for robotic surgery of the skull base. Laryngoscope. 2013;123(9):2176–9. https://doi.org/10.1002/lary.24034.
35. Dallan I, Castelnuovo P, Seccia V, Battaglia P, Montevecchi F, Tschabitscher M, Vicini C. Combined transnasal transcervical robotic dissection of posterior skull base: feasibility in a cadaveric model. Rhinology Journal. 2012;50(2):165–70. https://doi.org/10.4193/Rhin11.117.
36. Olaleye O, Jeong B, Switajewski M, Ooi EH, Krishnan S, Foreman A, Hodge J-C. Trans-oral robotic surgery for head and neck cancers using the Medrobotics flex® system: the Adelaide cohort. J Robot Surg. 2022;16(3):527–36. https://doi.org/10.1007/s11701-021-01270-z.
37. Brodie A, Vasdev N. The future of robotic surgery. Ann R Coll Surg Engl. 2018;100(Suppl 7):4–13. https://doi.org/10.1308/rcsann.supp2.4.

38. Revo-i competing on a par with Da Vinci. 2020. http://revosurgical.com/#/news_view.asp?B_Name=center&list_no=30&category=gallery
39. Gilbert H, Hendrick R, Remirez A, Webster R. A robot for transnasal surgery featuring needle-sized tentacle-like arms. Expert Rev Med Devices. 2014;11(1):5–7. https://doi.org/10.1586/17434440.2013.854702.
40. Swaney PJ, Gilbert HB, Iii RJW, Iii PTR, Weaver KD. Endonasal Skull Base tumor removal using concentric tube continuum robots: a phantom study. Journal of Neurological Surgery Part B: Skull Base. 2015;76(2):145–9. https://doi.org/10.1055/s-0034-1390401.
41. Bruns TL, Remirez AA, Emerson MA, Lathrop RA, Mahoney AW, Gilbert HB, Liu CL, Russell PT, Labadie RF, Weaver KD, Webster RJ. A modular, multi-arm concentric tube robot system with application to transnasal surgery for orbital tumors. The International Journal of Robotics Research. 2021;40(2–3):521–33. https://doi.org/10.1177/0278364921 1000074.
42. Chan JYK, Holsinger FC, Liu S, Sorger JM, Azizian M, Tsang RKY. Augmented reality for image guidance in transoral robotic surgery. J Robot Surg. 2020;14(4):579–83. https://doi.org/10.1007/s11701-019-01030-0.
43. Desai SC, Sung C-K, Genden EM. Transoral robotic surgery using an image guidance system. Laryngoscope. 2008;118(11):2003–5. https://doi.org/10.1097/MLG.0b013e3181818784.
44. Liu, W. P., Azizian, M., Sorger, J., Taylor, R. H., Reilly, B. K., Cleary, K., & Preciado, D. (2014). Cadaveric feasibility study of da Vinci Si–assisted Cochlear implant with augmented visual navigation for otologic surgery. *JAMA Otolaryngology–Head & Neck Surgery*, 140(3), 208–214. https://doi.org/10.1001/jamaoto.2013.6443.
45. Liu WP, Richmon JD, Sorger JM, Azizian M, Taylor RH. Augmented reality and cone beam CT guidance for transoral robotic surgery. J Robot Surg. 2015;9(3):223–33. https://doi.org/10.1007/s11701-015-0520-5.
46. Pratt P, Arora A. Transoral robotic surgery: image guidance and augmented reality. ORL. 2018;80(3–4):204–12. https://doi.org/10.1159/000489467.
47. Chicoine MR, Sylvester P, Yahanda AT, Shah A. Image guidance in cranial neurosurgery: how a six-ton magnet and fluorescent Colors make brain tumor surgery better. Mo Med. 2020;117(1):39–44.
48. Choi PJ, Oskouian RJ, Tubbs RS. Telesurgery: past, present, and future. Cureus. 2018;10(5):e2716. https://doi.org/10.7759/cureus.2716.
49. Mohan A, Wara UU, Shaikh MTA, Rahman RM, Zaidi ZA. Telesurgery and robotics: an improved and efficient era. Cureus. 2021;13(3) https://doi.org/10.7759/cureus.14124.
50. Kassahun Y, Yu B, Tibebu AT, Stoyanov D, Giannarou S, Metzen JH, Vander Poorten E. Surgical robotics beyond enhanced dexterity instrumentation: a survey of machine learning techniques and their role in intelligent and autonomous surgical actions. Int J Comput Assist Radiol Surg. 2016;11(4):553–68. https://doi.org/10.1007/s11548-015-1305-z.
51. Bhandari M, Zeffiro T, Reddiboina M. Artificial intelligence and robotic surgery: current perspective and future directions. Curr Opin Urol. 2020;30(1):48–54. https://doi.org/10.1097/MOU.0000000000000692.
52. CyberKnife—How it Works. (n.d.). CyberKnife. Retrieved May 31, 2022, from https://cyberknife.com/cyberknife-how-it-works/
53. Mako SmartRobotics Overview | Stryker. (n.d.). Retrieved May 31, 2022, from https://www.stryker.com/us/en/joint-replacement/systems/Mako_SmartRobotics_Overview.html#know-more
54. *Yomi Robotic System for dental implant surgery | Neocis Inc %.* (n.d.). Yomi By Neocis. Retrieved May 31, 2022, from https://www.neocis.com/
55. Iavazzo C, Gkegkes ID. Cost–benefit analysis of robotic surgery in gynaecological oncology. Best Pract Res Clin Obstet Gynaecol. 2017;45:7–18. https://doi.org/10.1016/j.bpobgyn.2017.03.008.

GPSR Compliance

The European Union's (EU) General Product Safety Regulation (GPSR) is a set of rules that requires consumer products to be safe and our obligations to ensure this.

If you have any concerns about our products, you can contact us on ProductSafety@springernature.com

In case Publisher is established outside the EU, the EU authorized representative is:

Springer Nature Customer Service Center GmbH
Europaplatz 3
69115 Heidelberg, Germany

Batch number: 10370712

Printed by Printforce, the Netherlands